614.
Z

WITHDRAWN FROM STOCK

prevent and control

in

Trust Library Services
North Manchester General Hospital
This item must be returned by the last
shown.
Renew by phone (0161 720 235?)
(NMGH.library@mft.nhs.uk)
Items can be renewed

L E ZIADY & N SMALL

In the writing of this book, every effort has been made to present accurate and up-to-date information from the best and most reliable sources. However, the results of nursing individuals depend on a variety of factors that are beyond the control of the authors and publishers. Therefore, neither the authors nor the publishers assume responsibility for, nor make any warranty as regards to, the outcomes achieved from the procedures described in this book.

First published as *Rapid Reference Infection Control* by Kagiso,
Paul Kruger Street, Pretoria. (ISBN 0-7986-4437-0)

Reprinted April 2006

© Juta and Co Ltd, 2004
PO Box 24309
Lansdowne 7779
Cape Town, South Africa

This book is copyright under the Berne Convention. In terms of the Copyright Act 98 of 1978, no part of this book may be reproduced or transmitted in any form or by any means, including photocopying, recording, or by any information storage and retrieval system, without permission in writing from the publisher.

ISBN 07021-6790-8

Project manager and editor: Sarah O'Neill
Proofreader: Andrew van der Spuy
Indexing: Andrew van der Spuy
Cover design: Christopher Davis
Designed and typeset in 10.5/13pt Minion and Franklin Gothic by Christopher Davis
Printed and bound in the Republic of South Africa by Paarl Print, Oosterland Street, Paarl

The authors and the publisher have made every effort to obtain permission for and acknowledge the use of copyright material. Should any infringement of copyright have occurred, please contact the publisher, and every effort will be made to rectify omissions or errors, in the event of a reprint or new edition.

This book is dedicated to the memory of Nico Small,
who passed away suddenly on 13th August 2004.
Dear friend, colleague and gentle giant, you are sorely missed.

Foreword

Infection control is a set of principles and guidelines which improve the quality and standard of patient care. In most developed countries, infection control programmes are an integral part of patient care in hospitals and the community. In the UK alone, hospital-acquired infections cost two billion pounds annually. Infection control is taken seriously indeed and full-time infection control teams (a doctor and nurse) are actively involved in reducing the burden of disease. In developing countries, infection control is of low priority and currently lacks adequate political support.

There is a dearth of books or reference material relevant to South Africa. The principal author – Laura Ziady – a well-established infection control nurse, has taken her extensive experience coupled with an in-depth literature review to produce a comprehensive guide to infection control. The book addresses infection control from a South African perspective, taking into account the multi-tasks an infection control practitioner faces in a working day. It contains advice on hospital and communicable disease control, with adequate explanation and rationale behind recommended practice.

Prevent and Control Infection: Application Made Easy is essential reading for anyone entering the arena of infection control, either as a student or tutor.

Prof. Shaheen Mehtar. MBBS, FRCPath (UK), FCPath (SA)
Head, Unit for Infection Control
Tygerberg Hospital and Stellenbosch University
Western Cape.

Contents

Chapter 3: Incident-related or hospital-acquired infections

SECTION 2: INFECTION CONTROL PRACTICE AND PROCEDURES

Chapter 4: Housekeeping

Chapter 5 : Disinfection and sterilisation

Chapter 6 : Clinical practice and procedures

Introduction

Why do we need infection control?

In the task-orientated world we live in, infection control is seen to be just another task that can be delegated to someone else. The truth is, however, that every person working in the healthcare environment is responsible for infection control. This task is not reserved for a specific healthcare worker or an Infection Control Department. Without a doubt, infection control is one of the primary functions of every person coming into contact with persons who are in need of care.

During the previous century, Florence Nightingale was reputed to have stated that 'The first requirement of any hospital is that it should do the sick no harm'. Do health care workers still adhere to this ideal? Today, iatrogenic (treatment-induced) disease seems to be a generally accepted side effect of hospitalisation.

The second requirement of healthcare settings is the protection of all who render a service against the risk of injury or disease. This is done through the availability of equipment and facilities. Guidelines for the management of patients and situations supplement the equipment and facilities. There is a need for staff to know how to protect and care for their patients and for themselves. As caregivers, we are taught that the patient is the most important person in a hospital, but we need to remember that we are just as important, if not more so.

Certain characteristics of healthcare settings promote the incidence of hospital acquired infection:

1. The **population** of these institutions, comprising:
   - Patients from different age groups. The very young and the elderly are usually less able to achieve or maintain a healthy resistance to infection. Age, disease, the level of expert care, immune suppression, medication and surgery all combine to make hospitals unhealthy places for the sick!
   - The number of patients cared for. Research has shown that when caregivers have a large number of patients to care for, then less time and attention is given to infection control practices.
2. High levels of **activity** and an active **flow of people, equipment, and provisions** in and out of wards and patient care areas are guaranteed to import more foreign and infectious micro-organisms into facilities.
3. **Technological development** has had good and bad consequences for healthcare. For example, few, if any, patient 'escapes' without having a blood sample taken, thus breaching the skin, one of the normal bodily defense mechanisms against infection.
4. The **unwise use of antibiotics and antiseptics** leads to the development of micro-organisms that are resistant to these compounds. The pathogens may even actively grow in weakened disinfectant solutions and attain a genetically acquired resistance. This leads to the development of **resistant strains of resident hospital pathogens** living and multiplying in the hospital environment.

Micro-organisms are part of the normal environment. No person or thing is free from them.

Usually humans live in symbiosis with most micro-organisms, but occasionally the micro-organisms become pathogenic and cause disease, due to a decline in the host's resistance, or an increased virulence or overwhelming growth of the microbe. Micro-organisms are always found in faeces, oral and sexual secretions, sputum, pus and wound drainage, and the urine of patients with catheters, and may be present in blood and urine other than from catheterised patients. Spillage, waste, wet equipment, the reuse of contaminated cleaning and disinfectant solutions and a soiled environment all encourage the proliferation of micro-organisms. These unseen opportunists are transferred through contact (directly from hand to surface, or indirectly through contamination of equipment and instruments); some are airborne in droplets or as nuclei in dust particles and others may be transmitted by vectors (insects) or vehicles such as blood and body fluids.

As opportunistic pathogens, micro-organisms penetrate the host's defense mechanisms, colonise the body and multiply. This results in a clinical host reaction. If control measures with human body fluid or blood are only implemented once a diagnosis is confirmed or an infection is suspected, it leads to double standards in patient care and the exposure of others to the infection.

The aim of infection control is to establish and maintain a safe environment for patients and staff members, providing the highest possible level of protection with the available resources, which should be aimed at real rather than theoretical hazards. The chain of infection requires a source of infection (a sick patient), a route of transfer (such as hands) and a new susceptible host. This chain needs to be broken in order to prevent the transmission of infection. If the route of infection is eliminated by hand-washing, the infection cannot be transferred.

Areas that require special attention for infection control include:

- Equipment that might have been in contact with contamination.
- Equipment that is used to invade normally sterile areas of the body.
- Articles used in specific contaminated patient-care areas or for invasive procedures.
- The immediate environment of patients with highly contagious or virulent conditions.
- The immediate environment of highly susceptible patients.

Standard infection control measures used in patient-care areas include destroying or removing pathogens or potential pathogens by means of general hygienic measures, good hand hygiene, and disinfection and sterilisation. Pathogens that cannot be destroyed or removed can usually be contained through the isolation of patients, the use of protective clothing, and the correct management of soiled or contaminated items. These measures are all elements of barrier nursing.

Ideally, control measures are aimed at providing a 'hostile environment' that prevents the multiplication of pathogens. A clean, dry and adequately ventilated patient-care area discourages colonisation by micro-organisms. Infection control measures also make provision for the protection of susceptible patients, staff and the environment, improved host resistance, the isolation and decontamination of infectious material and the identification of high-risk situations. Protective barriers must be used to prevent exposure of staff and patients to blood and human body fluid or substances such as tissue, excreta and secreta. These barriers must be appropriate for the procedure to be performed and the expected exposure to substances. Examples of protective barriers include gloves, waterproof aprons or gowns, masks, caps, eye protection (spectacles or goggles) and face shields.

In the subsequent sections, the following will be discussed:

Section 1: Micro-organisms
- Chapter 1: The relationship between micro-organisms and infection control practice
- Chapter 2: Disease-specific infection prevention and control measures
- Chapter 3: Incident-related or hospital-acquired infections

Section 2: Infection control and practice procedures
- Chapter 4: Housekeeping
- Chapter 5: Disinfection and sterilisation
- Chapter 6: Clinical practice and procedures
- Chapter 7: Special patient categories
- Chapter 8: Special issues
- Chapter 9: Staff issues
- Chapter 10: Infection control in home-based care settings

This reference guide is meant for use in all settings where the sick and helpless are seen or cared for, including rural or mobile clinics, hospitals and other patient-care areas. Chapters 2 and 3 of the guide can be used by healthcare practitioners and lay persons who require quick and summarised information on the best methods of infection control. Section 2 contains a discussion of some relevant patient care practices and suggested procedures with illustrations to highlight the more important facets thereof, as well as protocols that can be applied in practice. Chapter 10 is devoted to applying good infection control practice in the home environment.

The Infection Control Department: task description and placement in the hospital/ healthcare facility hierarchy

Objective

As stated previously, infection control is the responsibility of every staff member, but in order to ensure that correct infection control procedures are followed, it is necessary for management to establish a specific department, which will be responsible for the execution of all administrative aspects regarding prevention, identification and control of infection in the facility, as well as for specified delegated patient-care tasks, such as the isolation of cases of suspected formidable infectious diseases.

Functions

The main functions of the Infection Control Department consist of the following:
- Surveillance of infection control in the hospital/healthcare facility.
- Supervision of the execution of the hospital/healthcare facility policy on infection control as related to patient care, environmental hygiene and staff health.
- Formal and informal training and education, within the hospital/healthcare facility and in the greater outside community.
- Research.
- Liaison and communication with managers, staff and committees in the hospital/healthcare facility and the local health authority.
- Review of set policies or the creation of new policy and the appropriate infection control procedures, as well as the philosophy, objectives and goals of the department itself.
- Environmental monitoring.
- Medicine control and monitoring, as necessary, in co-operation with the medical microbiology laboratory and pharmacy.
- Liaison on staff health concerns with the Occupational Health Department, as necessary.
- Direct patient care in isolation for patients with suspected formidable diseases such as rabies or Crimean Congo viral haemorrhagic fever.
- Keeping records and statistics, and evaluation of data collected in this manner.

- Reporting as necessary on infection control practices and patient care.
- Notification to the local authorities, or the local or national Department of Health of legally notifiable diseases, as necessary.
- Consultation on infection control practices, or patient and staff health, and advice to the crèche, clinical laboratories, other disciplines and/or departments.
- Maintenance and support of the patient-directed quality improvement (assurance) programme of the facility.
- Monitoring the quality of the cleaning, disinfection, pasteurisation and sterilisation of reuseable items in the facility.
- Monitoring the quality of cleaning and environmental hygiene of the facility.
- Monitoring the quality of catering and food management.
- Executive membership of the Infection Control Committee of the facility.
- Active co-operation in the formal and informal training and education programmes of the facility.
- Orientation of all newly appointed nursing staff in infection control practice and principles.
- Attendance at meetings, symposia, conferences and other training opportunities.
- Active membership and representation on appropriate local and national associations regarding infection control matters.
- Counselling patients, staff or family members on aspects of isolation, infectious and contagious diseases and conditions.
- Research to collect new information.
- Evaluation, where appropriate, of procedures, equipment and supplies on different levels of infection control.
- Co-operation with other healthcare providers as and when requested by the hospital/healthcare facility management.
- Any other task as delegated by the direct supervisor or hospital/healthcare facility management.

- Membership of DORT (the Disease Outbreak Response Team programme of the local authority and/or region).

Objectives of infection control policies and procedures

The objectives of infection control policies and procedures are to set guidelines to prevent the spread of infections and contagious diseases, and to control and limit nosocomial (hospital-acquired) infections. They are:

- Prevention and/or control of the development and/or spread of contagious conditions/infection.
- Creation and maintenance of a hygienic and safe environment for patients, staff, visitors, the general public, as well as the community outside the hospital/healthcare facility.
- Giving guidance and setting guidelines for the isolation of patients or staff.
- Giving guidance and setting guidelines for the application of standard and universal preventive measures for the handling of blood and human body fluids, secretions, excretions, mucosa and non-intact skin.
- Functioning as consultant/reference source for inquiries from the community and other healthcare institutions and referring inquiries to the appropriate alternative sources.
- Training and formal education of individuals, groups and the community, e.g. medical students, pupil nurses and lay persons as well as healthcare staff from all categories and disciplines.
- Appropriate isolation of all patients with suspected or confirmed haemorrhagic diseases/formidable infectious conditions.

These infection control policies and procedures are applicable to all persons present on the hospital/healthcare facility's premises, including staff, patients, voluntary workers, student learners or trainees, the general public and any private service provider's workers.

Responsibility

- The chief executive officer of the facility is responsible for the implementation and execution of the infection control policies and procedures, with the assistance of the Infection Control Department.
- The Infection Control Department reports to the Infection Control Committee – both in writing and verbally – on incidents, surveillance programmes, interventions and changes in infection control practices.
- All staff must be informed regularly about the infection control programme and procedures during orientation programmes and in-service training.
- A written infection control guide containing the policy and procedures must be supplied to each patient-care area.
- Staff are responsible and accountable for delivery of service within the parameters of the set policy.

Acceptance and delivery of policy

The chief executive officer accepts or declines the preliminary policy and procedures for the prevention and control of contagious diseases and infection on behalf of hospital/healthcare facility management, in accordance with the needs and functional necessity of the institution. He is also responsible for initiating a method by which the set policy can be made effective.

Responsibilities and accountability of the Infection Control Department and staff

Responsibility and authority over infection control practice is delegated to the appropriate staff on different levels of the hospital/ healthcare facility. The persons to whom responsibility and authority have been delegated are accountable for their own acts and omissions, as well as for those of the staff under their supervision.

Procedure

The healthcare facility's chief executive officer delegates administrative authority, responsibility and accountability for the implementation of the facility's infection control programme and procedures to the Infection Control Department and Committee. The Infection Control Committee has the responsibility to determine if effective prevention and control measures have been implemented to prevent, evaluate or control any outbreaks or incidents of infection in the hospital/ healthcare facility.

The division of responsibility and accountability for infection control in the healthcare facility is as detailed below.

Hospital/healthcare facility management responsibilities

The hospital/healthcare facility management is responsible for ensuring that:
- Appropriate and adequate measures are taken to control hospital infections by appointing an Infection Control Committee and infection control staff.
- The recommendations of the committee are implemented and executed.
- An Occupational Health and Safety Committee is appointed to deal in part with staff health issues and to make certain that attention is given to any complaints or recommendations that the committee may make.
- The hospital/healthcare facility's functions are executed in a safe environment to protect staff, patients, visitors and other persons as far as possible against exposure to, and development of, infection.

- No person suffering from a highly transmittable condition is appointed, e.g. a carrier of typhoid. Carriers of less contagious conditions such as HIV, or treatable infections, e.g. drug-resistant *Staphylococcus aureus* infection must initially be placed in areas where there is a minimal risk of spread of the condition to other staff members or patients. After discussion with the individual and careful review of the situation by the Occupational Health Department, the appointment or placement of a person with a diagnosed, treatable condition may be delayed until treatment has commenced and/or the condition has cleared up.
- Immunisation is available against vaccine-preventable diseases, and is utilised as far as possible.
- Facilities are available where infected patients can be cared for with the minimum of risk for transfer of the condition, utilising reasonable preventive measures that include isolation.
- Access of any visitor with a known contagious condition that can spread to patients and staff is limited in an appropriate manner to prevent cross-infection.
- Infection is not spread to others due to the discharge of patients with contagious conditions.
- Staff maintain the highest possible standards of aseptic technique and hygiene to prevent the infection of patients.
- All functional measures are implemented as far as possible for the safe handling, use, storage, and transport of articles and agents generated or used in the healthcare setting, to protect and minimise the risk to the health of the staff.
- Safety Committees are appointed to look into specific aspects of staff health or to investigate incidents.
- Protective barriers, clothing and personal protection equipment are available at all times to protect both patients and staff against infection.
- Infection control, surveillance, audit and quality assurance programmes are implemented and maintained.
- All staff take part in infection prevention and control programmes.

Infection Control Committee responsibilities

The Infection Control Committee is responsible and accountable for:
- Setting standards to provide and maintain a safe and infection-free environment.
- Recommending measures to resolve current and/or potential problems.
- Lowering the risk of hospital-acquired infections and the potential for infections for patients, staff, the community and the environment through the establishment and maintenance of preventative and epidemiologically indicated precautions, as well as the notification and management of infections.
- Implementing, monitoring and evaluating policies to guide the infection control programme.
- Implementing set policy by ensuring that staff have the necessary authority and resources to enforce it, and thereby ensuring the co-operation of all staff.
- Co-ordinating and ensuring the co-operation of different expert departments during the management and/or control of outbreaks of infection.
- Identifying and correcting risky and/or inefficient infection control procedures.
- Ensuring that the different members of the committee have the necessary expertise in decision making and problem solving.

Infection Control Committee

The Infection Control Committee should consist of the following people:

- chief executive officer of the healthcare setting or a delegated representative
- adjunct nursing service manager or a delegated representative
- infection control staff
- medical microbiologist(s)
- medical virologist(s)
- catering service representative
- pharmacy staff
- occupational health staff
- representatives from the main medical disciplines in the healthcare setting
- any other person needed to serve on the committee on an ad hoc or more permanent basis.

The Infection Control Committee appoints a day management team that takes care of the day-to-day problems of the healthcare facility and meets every month, e.g. the infection control practitioner and a medical microbiologist. The agenda and minutes of meetings should be circulated to all relevant disciplines. At least one full committee meeting should be convened twice annually, to which all concerned persons and interested parties are invited. All suggested discussion points for the agenda must reach the secretary at least one week before the set date of the next meeting.

Infection Control Officer

The responsibilities and accountability of the Infection Control Officer (nurse specialist or physician) include:
- Membership of the day management of the Infection Control Committee.
- Monitoring of infections and methods of control, speedy identification and investigation of outbreaks or potentially dangerous procedures.
- Assessment of the risk of infection.
- Advice on isolation of infected patients or the control of the spread of infection.
- Supervision of suggested measures in all patient-care areas of the hospital/healthcare facility.
- Consultation, co-ordination and co-operation with all disciplines of medical staff in the hospital/healthcare facility.
- Supply of information and advice on clinical patient care.
- Liaison with medical microbiology and virology laboratories as well as other clinical patient service laboratory services.
- Liaison with the infection control nursing staff delegated to patient-care areas.
- Assessment of the need for and use of environmental monitoring, e.g. laboratory analysis of milk feeds for paediatric and critical care patients, or water from municipal reservoirs.
- Implementation of the decisions of the Infection Control Committee or adjustment of policy if necessary.
- Continued personal study and technical development.
- Any additional responsibility on request of the hospital/healthcare facility management or the Infection Control Committee.
- Research, e.g. regarding new products introduced to the Infection Control Committee.

Infection control nursing staff

The responsibilities and accountability of the infection control nursing staff include:
- Knowledge of all the disciplines and functional departments in the healthcare facility.
- Regular contact with the patient-care areas.
- Training staff from all departments regarding infection control policy and procedures.
- Evaluation of set policy for efficiency, appropriateness and practicality so that it may be reviewed and updated if found inadequate.
- Advising, consulting and performing as a source of reference where necessary.
- Supplying formal and informal education and training to all disciplines of staff and workers in the healthcare setting.

- Running surveillance programmes in the healthcare setting.
- Keeping statistics and records.
- Investigating infection outbreaks and evaluating set interventions and infection control measures/barriers.
- Supervising patient-care procedures, staff health and environmental hygiene, where appropriate.
- Supervising staff who are nursing patients in isolation.
- Observing quality management and consultation where possible.
- Liaison with the hospital/healthcare facility management, supervisors of patient-care areas, and training staff on the care of patients with hospital- or community-acquired infection.
- Assistance with the evaluation of sterilisation, disinfection and cleaning procedures in the hospital.
- Assistance with the identification of routes and sources of cross-infection in patient-care areas.
- Presentation of infection control problems to the Infection Control Officer, the Infection Control Committee or the hospital/healthcare facility management as they occur.
- Attending in-service training courses, continuous education, seminars and congresses to update knowledge and expertise.
- Transfer of knowledge gained as discussed under the previous point.
- Preparation of reports as requested by the healthcare facility, local or national Department of Health, the Occupational Health and Safety Committee, or any other source.
- Liaison with all patient-care areas and support services, e.g. the pharmacy, catering service, laundry and cleaning service.
- Identification of potential risks and the presentation of measures to control or prevent infection.

- Liaison on patients' infectious conditions with the medical microbiology and virology laboratories.
- Speedy notification to the appropriate authorities of formidable, highly infectious or contagious diseases.
- Membership of appropriate committees.
- Research.
- Any other responsibilities as requested by the hospital/healthcare facility management or Infection Control Committee.

Other hospital/healthcare facility staff

The responsibilities and accountability of other hospital/healthcare facility staff rest on their professional acts and omissions, patient-care skills and the manner in which the facility's set policy and procedures are executed. All staff should be aware of the following points:

- Infection control (personal and patient-orientated) is the individual responsibility of each staff member who supplies direct or indirect patient care in the hospital/healthcare facility, as well as the responsibility of patients who know that they are suffering from infection.
- Each registered nurse is responsible for the acts of staff under his/her supervision, as well as the safe infection control practices of all who work in that patient-care area, e.g. doctors, students and paramedical staff such as physiotherapists. The senior staff member on duty has the right to insist on safe patient-care practices, such as handwashing and disinfection, for the sake of both the patients and the staff.
- The professional nurse supervisor of a patient-care area is responsible for ensuring the availability of necessary protective clothing and equipment, such as plastic bags, soap and towels or disinfectant (or appropriate replacements) in the area. If this is not done, documented (written) evidence must be produced to show that no supplies were available/issued by the stores

or another supplier (e.g. requisitions marked 'No supply available', as well as a note that the matter was reported to the appropriate nursing service manager).

- The professional nurse supervisor of a patient-care area must ensure that he/she, as well as the rest of the staff in that area, are in possession of sufficient knowledge to implement and maintain infection control in the ward. If not, he/she should imple-ment steps to correct any deficit.

- Each patient-care area must have an official institutional infection control guide available so that staff can avail themselves of information as necessary. If the necessary information is not available in the patient-care area, or additional information is required, the staff should contact the Infection Control Department for assistance.

Section One
Micro-organisms

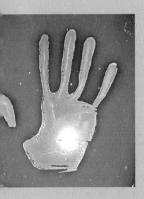

Chapter 1   The relationship between micro-organisms and infection control practice

Chapter 2   Disease-specific infection prevention and control measures

Chapter 3   Incident-related or hospital-acquired infections

In Section 1, the interface between the human host and the 'visitors' from the invisible world of micro-organisms is discussed. Some of the more common commensal and pathogenic micro-organisms are listed, while disease-specific infection prevention and control measures are suggested in cases where the pathogen is known to the healthcare staff. This is done as a summary of conditions in chapter 2 and in an overview of measures in chapter 3, in order to accommodate those situations where healthcare staff do not (yet) have a laboratory or clinically defined diagnosis for the patient's assessed condition, but prevention and control measures are indicated.

The Center for Disease Control and Prevention (CDC) in Atlanta, Georgia, USA is recognised as one of the leading authorities in the field of infection control. The Web site at www.cdc.gov offers further information on the conditions dealt with in chapters 2 and 3.

1 | The relationship between micro-organisms and infection control practice

Introduction

We live in a world of potential infection. The human being and his living and non-living environment carry a multitude of micro-organisms that may cause one or more infections, depending on circumstances and opportunity. Humans in particular are a constant reservoir (source) of micro-organisms, which can vary and change as a person comes into contact with new and old environments, other people, animals and materials. During different times of the day we carry differing 'biological loads' and numbers of viable micro-organisms.

The human body is naturally colonised with micro-organisms and the presence thereof does not necessarily mean infection is present or that treatment is indicated. (Refer to chapter 6, page 190 on specimen collection.)

Organisms that cause infection are described as pathogens. Other organisms that would under normal circumstances not cause infection are classified as non-pathogenic or commensal organisms. An organism that may be accepted as a commensal on one part of the body, such as staphylococcus on an intact skin, may well cause an opportunistic infection if it should be deposited on a wound surface. Commensal organisms usually live in symbiosis with the host, to the benefit of both.

Types of micro-organisms

Between 5–15% of all patients admitted to hospitals develop a hospital-acquired infection (HAI), caused by one or more of the four main types of micro-organisms. These four traditional types of micro-organisms are all microscopic in size, and though they cannot be seen with the naked eye, they act as opportunistic pathogens if circumstances allow.

Protozoa are the largest of the living micro-organisms and can reach 0,1 mm in size. These microbes usually causes localised infections. The main protozoal infections include trichomoniasis, amoebic dysentry, giardiasis and malaria. Giardiasis often presents in crèches and play-groups where children are crowded together and faecal-oral transfer soon takes place. Specific anti-protozoal medication is necessary to fight these micro-organisms.

Fungi are the second-largest type of living micro-organism and are commonly encountered in the infection of immune-compromised patients such as neonates, HIV-positive patients, asthmatic and critical-care patients, as well as those persons with metabolic abnormalities such as diabetes. Patients on long-term broad-spectrum antibiotics are prone to an overgrowth of fungal infections when their normal bacteria start dying off due to the antibiotic(s). The most common fungal infections include candidiasis (thrush), aspergillosis, ringworm, fungal meningitis and athlete's foot. Specific anti-fungal medication is indicated to fight fungal infection.

Bacteria are the third-largest type of living micro-organism and the most commonly encountered because of their wide dispersion in the environment. Some species of bacteria are able to divide every 20 minutes. One bacterium can multiply into 100 million in 10 hours, in temperatures of between 6°C and

60°C. Some types prefer oxygen-rich environments (aerobic species) or oxygen-poor environments (anaerobic species). All organisms need moistness to grow, and die down in dry conditions. Food is another important requirement, although some species can remain viable for long periods with the minimum of nutrition.

Bacteria are classified into four basic forms, namely.

- (long) rods
- (round) cocci
- (spirals) spirochete, and
- (wave-like) vibrios.

Some bacteria have additional characteristics such as:

- flagella that help propel them through fluids
- capsules that assist them to survive for long periods in inhospitable environments, and
- spore formation, which ensures that the micro-organisms will withstand disinfectants as well as long periods of drought.

Pathogenic bacteria are especially protected by the particular characteristics or structures they often display.

Bacteria are further classified into two main groups by Gram-staining in a laboratory. After staining, Gram-positive bacteria show up blue under the microscope, while Gram-negative organisms colour red. In hospitals the Gram-negative micro-organisms are usually more of a problem to eradicate, although some of the Gram-positive organisms are becoming as difficult to treat.

The tubercle bacteria that cause tuberculosis are more resistant to disinfectants than many other vegetative (growing) micro-organisms. They can survive relatively well in droplets and remain viable for quite long periods in dust. Specific antibiotics are required to treat each specific bacterial infection.

Viruses are the smallest form of micro-organism, and are defined as active or passive rather than living or dead. Some pathogenic viruses are regularly encountered during outbreaks of hospital-acquired infection such as herpes, chicken pox, measles, hepatitis, HIV, polio, rotavirus, influenza or colds. The virus multiplies inside the host's cells and is usually passive when separated from the host. Transfer of viruses requires reasonably close contact between the source of infection and the new susceptible host (e.g. contact with contaminated hands of a sick person, or a needle prick is needed to transmit hepatitis or HIV).

Treatment of viral infections is difficult because the virus is present in the form of particles in the cells. Often during treatment the treated host's uninfected cells are destroyed at the same time as the infected ones. Hepatitis B is prone to forming spores that remain viable on surfaces for long periods and are heat resistant. Practically all respiratory diseases and childhood ailments are viral, with bacteria as a second cause. Only specific anti-viral medications are effective against viral infections.

Prions are infectious proteins and not traditional micro-organisms as such, which cause disorders such as Creutzfeld-Jakob disease and 'mad cow' disease. These are starting to present more often in individual and epidemic format. Medical science does not presently have any way to combat them.

Definition of an infection

Infection is the penetration and multiplication of an infectious micro-organism in or on a new, susceptible host's body, followed by a clinically observed reaction.

The sources of infection

There are two main sources of infection:
- Endogenous infection, also known as self-

infection. The source of infection is the patient him- or herself. When the body's normal defence mechanism is breached, e.g. after massive trauma where the skin and tissue are damaged, normal commensal micro-organisms may become opportunistic pathogens. Most endogenous infection is caused by micro-organisms from the patient's intestinal tract or skin.

- Exogenous infection, also called cross-infection. This is caused by micro-organisms from outside the patient's body. Staff, other patients, or a contaminated environment may be the source of this type of infection.

Transmission routes of infection

Micro-organisms are transferred from one patient to another, or from one patient to the staff and/or the environment, by four main methods:

1. Direct contact between the source of infection and the susceptible host or go-between. An important method of transfer is the hands of staff, as they have direct contact with patients, colleagues and the environment during the course of their normal duties.
2. Indirect contact takes place when a patient or staff member contaminates an item and the micro-organisms are transferred from this item to a second person or the environment, and then to a susceptible host. Example: an infected patient's toy falls on the contaminated floor, which already carries micro-organisms from all the staff moving around and patients playing on the floor of that room. Someone picks up the contaminated toy, in turn contaminating their hands, and returns it, unwashed, to the child. The helper's hands are contaminated directly and the patient indirectly through the toy.
3. Vectors are insects that carry micro-organisms from one host to another, e.g. malaria-infected mosquitoes bite a non–infected human host, and transfer the infecting protozoa in this manner.
4. Airborne transmission takes place where drops of mucus are set free in the air when a person talks, coughs or shouts. Large drops quickly settle on the ground but smaller ones float around as aerosols that cling to dust particles. The fluid part of the drop evaporates and the pathogens become part of the circulating dust. This dust takes a long time to settle and can infect the environment and any unprotected and/or susceptible surface in the process.

Some common types of infection

Key to the chart:
CAI = Community-acquired infection.
HAI = Hospital-acquired infection.

Table 2a: Fungal infections

Types of infection	Disease	Mode of transmission	Infection
Candida albicans	Candida of the mouth, gastrointestinal tract, genitalia, bacteraemia, thrombophlebitis, endocarditis.	Contact with contaminated hands, equipment, poor aseptic technique, endogenous infection from gastrointestinal tract.	CAI or HAI
Aspergillus species	Aspergillus food poisoning.	Airborne, contact with contaminated hands and equipment.	CAI or HAI

Table 2b: Parasitic infections

Types of infection	Disease	Mode of transmission	Infection
Cryptosporidium	Diarrhoea.	Contact with stool from animals or birds or contaminated water.	CAI
Toxoplasmosis gondi	Foetal abnormalities in the first trimester, cerebral toxoplasmosis in HIV patients.	Contact with the faeces of cats and other infected animals, transplanted organs, ingestion of raw or partially cooked meat.	CAI or HAI
Plasmodium	Malaria.	Contact with blood containing the parasite, bite of an infected mosquito, unscreened blood transfusion, contaminated needles and syringes.	CAI or HAI

Table 2c: Bacteria/Gram-positive cocci

Types of infection	Disease	Mode of transmission	Infection
Staphylococcus aureus	Skin infection, e.g. abscesses and wounds.	Contact with exudates and hands, also airborne.	CAI or HAI
Staphylococcus epidermidis	Central venous catheter sepsis, endocarditis, bacteraemia.	Contact with hands and skin flakes.	CAI or HAI
Enterococcus	Urinary tract or wound infection, endocarditis.	Contact with hands, dust, skin flakes, cross-infection.	CAI or HAI
Streptococcus pyogenes	Necrotising fasciitis, sore throat, tonsillitis, cellulitis, impetigo, septicaemia, scarlet fever.	Contact with hands, droplet contamination, contaminated fomites.	CAI or HAI

Table 2d: Bacteria/Gram-negative cocci

Types of infection	Disease	Mode of transmission	Infection
Neisseria gonorrhoea	Urethritis (males), vaginitis (females), arthritis, dermatitis, ophthalmia neonatorum.	Sexual contact, contact during normal delivery.	CAI or HAI

Table 2e: Bacteria/Gram-positive bacilli

Types of infection	Disease	Mode of transmission	Infection
Bacillus cereus	Food poisoning.	Ingestion of contaminated food, contact with contaminated hands, contamination of infusion wounds.	CAI or HAI
Clostridium perfringens	Skin and soft tissue infection, septic abortion, food poisoning.	Contact with contaminated soil or hands or ingestion of contaminated food.	CAI or HAI

Table 2f: Bacteria/Gram-negative bacilli

Types of infection	Disease	Mode of transmission	Infection
Pseudomonas aeruginosa	Urinary tract infection, intravenous catheter sepsis, infected wounds and burns.	Contact with contaminated water, contaminated disinfectants, humidifiers, droplet transmission.	CAI or HAI
Acinetobacter baumannii, Acinetobacter species	Infection of wounds, the urinary and respiratory tracts, septicaemia.	Contact with contaminated hands, contaminated solutions, skin flakes and droplet transmission, and contamination of intravenous lines.	CAI or HAI
Vibrio cholerae	Cholera.	Faecal-oral transmission, contact with contaminated hands, water, food and flies.	CAI or HAI
Shigella species	Shigellosis (diarrhoea).	Faecal-oral transmission, contact with contaminated water, food, hands and flies.	CAI or HAI
Salmonella typhi	Typhoid fever.	Faecal-oral transmission, contact with contaminated water, food, hands and flies.	CAI or HAI
Klebsiella pneumoniae, Klebsiella species	Pneumonia, wound infection and infection of the urinary tract, bacteraemia.	Contact with contaminated hands, infusion fluid and equipment.	CAI or HAI

16

Sepsis/asepsis

The objective of infection control is to ensure that all articles needed for direct patient care, as well as the environment itself, are aseptic/clean and carry a low bioload (as few micro-organisms as possible) to ensure safety. This includes surfaces that have been in contact with micro-organisms, which are also seen as contaminated.

Definitions

Sepsis is a systemic disease caused by the presence of pathogens, pyogens and other micro-organisms with their toxin in the patient's tissues and bloodstream.

Septicaemia is the presence of pathogenic bacteria and toxin in the patient's blood.

Asepsis is the absence of pathogen micro-organisms.

- Medical asepsis indicates the measures that are utilised to prevent micro-organisms from surviving, growing, multiplying and spreading, e.g. barrier nursing.
- Surgical asepsis consists of the measures that are utilised in an operation theatre to prevent/control the development and spread of infection.

Aseptic technique is the procedure(s) utilised to prevent the transfer or spread of micro-organisms.

Disinfection is the removal or inactivation of vegetative micro-organisms on surfaces, excluding bacterial spores.

Pasteurisation is the use of moist heat/heating between 65–90°C to destroy vegetative micro-organisms.

Sterilisation is the destruction of all living micro-organisms and spores.

Using protective clothing and equipment, such as plastic bags and sharps containers, is one method of medical asepsis devised to contain micro-organisms (barrier nursing).

The patient and everything in his/her environment that he/she touches will become a source of micro-organisms. As a result the measures utilised for infection prevention and control are mutually inclusive and all-embracing.

Aseptic procedures include the management of linen, waste, equipment, sharps, visitors, staff, occupational health, patient-care procedures and environmental hygiene. All health education includes aspects of asepsis.

Legal notification of contagious/infectious diseases

Discussion

By law, a number of conditions have been classed as legally notifiable, some due to their infectiousness/risk of transmission, and some to evaluate the health status of the community or to give warning that immunisation programmes are not functioning sufficiently. You will find a list of notifiable diseases in appendix 1 on page 248–9. This list of conditions is periodically updated and published by the Minister of Health in the Government Gazette.

In order that timely and appropriate precautionary measures are taken, the Infection Control Department must be notified of all infectious/transmissible conditions, especially those specified by law. The initial notification is by telephone after diagnosis/admittance.

The treating doctor or registered nurse in charge of the case must report all notifiable diseases in writing as soon as possible after confirmation of diagnosis. The GW 17/5 form must contain a residential address (street address) and be sent to the Infection Control Department, from where it will be sent to the appropriate local authority. An example of form GW 17/5 is included on page 115.

In the case of different types of food poisoning, certain conditions for notification are found: if **four or more** patients from the same source of poisoning are admitted/treated, it is considered to be an outbreak of food poisoning and becomes notifiable by the attending doctor.

Rabies, meningococcal meningitis and viral haemorrhagic fevers are the exceptions: as soon as the suspected diagnosis is made, the attending doctor must contact the Infection Control Department, the patient's own referring physician and the Deputy Director of Communicable Diseases in the local Department of Health, so that the tracing of contacts may begin. As soon as the diagnosis is confirmed, the telephonic message is followed in writing by the GW 17/5 written notification from the attending doctor.

The Infection Control Department will assist the patient-care area with advice on the isolation measures necessary to protect the patient and the staff, if necessary.

Any case of infection that develops after the patient has been hospitalised for 48 hours or longer must be investigated as a hospital-acquired infection (HAI). Patients that are admitted with infectious diseases or who have contagious conditions must also be reported to the Infection Control Department, so that measures may be taken in time to prevent the spread of the condition to other patients or staff.

Management principles and measures to control and prevent infection and maintain asepsis

Also consult the section on standard infection prevention and control precautions in chapter 6, page 171.

Hand-washing and hygiene

Hand-washing is the single most important preventative/control measure against the spread of infection. Hands should be washed:

- Before and after contact with the patient, his/her direct environment (i.e. the bed, locker), excretions, secretions, and all organic material such as blood, body fluids or body tissue.
- Before and after the use of gloves.

Procedure

- Hands must be washed for at least 30–60 seconds using the appropriate soap and following the correct procedure by applying enough friction and washing under running water. Also consider the reason for the wash (social wash for 30 seconds, or aseptic scrub for an initial 60 seconds).
- Special consideration should be given to washing the palms and the back of the hands, between the fingers, the sides of the hand and the fingertips as these are the areas that usually receive least attention.
- Rubbing removes as many transient micro-organisms from the skin folds as soap and water, enabling the running water to rinse away the micro-organisms. Complete the process by drying with a paper towel.
- If the water should splash over the basin and onto the clothes of the person washing, the environment becomes contaminated with the organisms from the hands. Cross-infection may follow.
- The first scrub for an aseptic technique, such as a surgical operation, must last at least one minute to clean the skin effectively.
- Hands and other skin surfaces are washed if contaminated items are handled or if hands are soiled with human blood, body fluid or tissue.
- Hands must be washed before gloves are put on and after they are removed, even if it appears as if the gloves are intact, as the skin perspires under the glove and more normal micro-organisms are released from the hair follicles and skin pores.

Hand-drying

The use of paper towels to dry washed hands is the most hygienic method available as they are used once and then discarded. Friction from the paper towel removes another layer of transient micro-organisms from the skin. Cotton or linen towels rapidly become a source of contamination as they allow micro-organisms to multiply on damp and soiled surfaces. A dry environment is less hospitable to micro-organisms, which causes them to die off quickly. Hot-air dryers circulate huge counts of micro-organisms that are then deposited on the washed hands. This type of drying is so time-consuming that most staff members do not wait for their hands to dry completely before rushing off. Cross-infection is thus encouraged by the use of hot-air dryers.

Hand disinfection

- Hand disinfection is always indicated before and after contact with the patient, his/her direct environment (i.e. bed and locker), as long as there is no overt soiling of hands with organic material. In cases where the hands are visibly soiled they should be washed, because application of disinfectant over organic material deactivates the chemical ingredients.
- Hands that have been disinfected before putting on unsterile gloves for a non-aseptic procedure are better protected as gloves are not always impermeable.
- Disinfection before entering and after leaving the room of a patient in isolation (either direct or reversed isolation) ensures (added) protection for both staff members and patients.
- A mixture of alcohol and disinfectant with glycerin (to prevent excess drying of hands) or a commercial product should be supplied in spray bottles that can be manipulated by the user's elbow. 3–8 ml of the solution is sprayed into the palm of the hand and rubbed over the surface of both hands until dry. Special attention should be paid to the fingertips, palms and sides, between the fingers and the back of the hands. The process may be repeated between patient care procedures/patient contact until the hands become sticky from the emollient. Washing with soap and water is then appropriate. Try to avoid products containing liquid paraffin as an emollient, as this is more difficult to remove from the skin with washing and tends to protect skin micro-organisms, which remain under the applied layer.

Single room

Indicated for use

- When the patient is suffering from or may suffer from an airborne infectious disease.
- When the patient is unable to maintain good personal hygiene.
- When the patient has an infectious condition caused by a drug-resistant micro-organism or organisms (microbes resistant to antibiotics).
- When the patient has an infection that carries a high risk of environmental contamination.
- When the patient has an underlying condition that makes him/her more susceptible to a health-threatening cross-infection from the environment, other patients or staff members (i.e. leukaemic patients in protective isolation).
- When the patient is terminally ill.

Instructions for use

- Where possible the door of the protective isolation room must remain closed (the patient is to be protected against infection from external sources).
- The hands **must** be disinfected before entering and after leaving the room.

- The door of a room where the patient is in direct isolation can be left open and should only be kept closed if the patient has an airborne infection. (Direct or source isolation protects other patients and staff from exposure to an infection).

Plastic aprons/impermeable aprons

Indicated for use

- When the clothes/uniform of the healthcare worker may become contaminated or soiled with organic material, such as human tissue or body fluids (blood, faeces or urine).
- During physical contact with the patient, e.g. when small children are carried or held on the lap of staff members.
- Whilst performing certain aseptic procedures, i.e. extensive wound care, or if the staff member needs to support him- or herself against the bed to turn a patient.
- When handling contaminated/soiled articles or equipment (e.g. bed linen).
- When organisms from the skin of the healthcare worker, the environment or other patients pose a threat of infection to the patient (such as during protective isolation of an immunosuppressed patient).
- Where dual protection is needed to prevent contamination between patients and staff members.

Instructions for use

- Plastic aprons may be used repeatedly for a round of wound care procedures or for a period of time whilst caring for a single patient.
- Disinfect or wash the outside of the apron between procedures/patient contact to prevent transfer of contamination/soiling. The apron can be disinfected by soaking a paper towel in disinfectant and then wiping the entire surface of the apron. Micro-organisms are removed by a combination of disinfectant and friction. Spraying disinfectant directly onto the apron is ineffective: disinfecting is only effective when combined with the rubbing/wiping motion. Aprons can then be hung just inside the door to the patient's room so that they may be donned before approaching the patient. Aprons must be hung separately (not on top of each other) so that unnoticed contamination/soiling is not transferred from one to the other.

- Aprons for reuse must be marked on the outside with the date so that they may be replaced every 24 hours whilst the outside – which carries the potential of contaminating the wearer's own clothes – is readily identifiable. The surface of an apron deteriorates from regular disinfecting and the resulting roughness may harbour micro-organisms.
- If an apron is to be discarded, it should be disinfected for the last time to remove all contamination and then destroyed by tearing it up. This prevents another person from using a contaminated apron.
- Store new, unused aprons where they cannot be contaminated/soiled by accident.

Gloves

Indicated for use

- When carrying out sterile aseptic procedures to protect the patient from infection.
- During unsterile procedures where the staff must be protected from infection/contamination.
- Where the hands of healthcare workers pose an infection risk to susceptible patients (e.g. immunosuppressed patients).

Instructions for use

- Sterile or unsterile disposable gloves are used depending on the requirements of the procedure to be done. Soiled, gloved hands may be washed at least once or twice while working with one patient. Alcohol and soap cause gloves to corrode, become sticky and harbour micro-organisms in the roughened surface. Disposable gloves should not be reused. When removing gloves, they must be turned inside out and discarded before washing hands to rid hands of perspiration and glove powder. Unseen contamination may penetrate the glove through microscopic pinholes in the material.

- Gloves should be changed after every 2 hours of continuous use, or when they become sticky or perforated. Gloves contribute to large-scale environmental contamination if used incorrectly.
- Gloves must be removed and discarded before leaving the patient's room – staff members must avoid wandering around passages and store rooms wearing gloves.
- Containers of unused, new gloves should be kept where they cannot be contaminated by accident, and where a person removing one glove cannot soil/contaminate the others.
- Never assume that gloves provide 100% protection against all infections. The manufacturing process may cause microscopic pinholes in the glove where the material is thinner. These areas may perforate when the glove is in use. Stretching the material forms a small vacuum where pathogens may be sucked into the glove. Micro-organisms on the wearer's hand may also be expelled through the pinhole.

Surgical face masks

Indicated for use

- For contact with patients with airborne infections – though the caregiver should maintain a distance of at least one meter where possible.
- Where the staff member's airway, nose, throat or other mucosa may be exposed to organic material such as droplets, splashes or splatters of blood, sputum or other body fluids.
- Where the susceptible patient may be threatened by airborne micro-organisms originating from the staff member (e.g. immunosuppressed patients).

Instructions for use

- Only surgical filter-type masks with a built-in filter are safe. Other masks are more permeable and allow droplets and microbes in aerosols through. These masks endanger the patient rather than protecting him/her.
- Masks must cover the nose and mouth completely – anything less is a waste of time and effort.
- All the ties must be fastened so that the mask follows the natural curve of the jawline. Air must escape from the sides of the mask and not from the bottom as this blows over the wearer's work area and hands.
- The metal nose bridge of the mask must fit properly over the nose (and, where indicated, under the spectacles) of the wearer.
- Masks are disposable and should be used only once and then discarded. Handle masks by the ties only. **Never** leave masks hanging around the neck or place a used mask in a pocket for re-use. This promotes contamination of the clothes with organisms from the wearer's airways and the environment.
- Hands must be washed before masks are donned as well as after removal, to prevent contamination of clean masks or from used ones.
- Avoid touching the mask unnecessarily, as this may contaminate the mask or hands.
- Masks should be stored in dustproof containers so that the possibility of contamination is eliminated.
- High-particulate filter (e.g. N95) masks can be used in situations where the staff must remain by the patient's bedside and the patient has a formidable contagious infection

such as severe acute respiratory syndrome ('SARS') or multi-drug-resistant tuberculosis.

- Masks should be replaced after two hours of continuous use or as soon as they become damp.

Caps/head protection

Indicated for use

- During aseptic procedures, or other tasks when there is a risk of contamination of the hair with splatter or splashes of drops/aerosols from patients. Caps also protect the patient from contamination with microbes or skin flakes from the staff member's hair and head. Hair carries a full complement of a person's normal skin flora, only in far greater numbers than the hands, which are washed more often.
- During protective isolation, where the patient is susceptible to infection, i.e. after bone marrow transplants or with leukaemia patients on chemotherapy. For an immunosuppressed patient, the normal skin flora of another person poses a real threat to life and recovery.

Instructions for use

- Caps must completely cover the hair up to the hairline.
- Hands must be washed or disinfected before and after handling caps to minimise the risk of contamination.
- Avoid unnecessarily touching the cap to prevent contamination of it or of the hands.
- Caps must be removed and discarded before leaving the patient's room, and as soon as they become damp/soiled/torn. Perspiration or splatters of aerosols/droplets cause contamination of caps that may be transferred to the hair, the environment or the patient via the wearer's hands. Because of this, disposable caps are never reused.

- When donning or removing a cap, it must be handled by the elastic or outer edge only. This is because the wearer's hair has contaminated the inside of the cap, and the outside has been contaminated by dust or organic matter from the procedure/patient.
- Caps must be stored in a covered container where no unauthorised person has access to them and contamination is avoided. Contamination of clean supplies may necessitate that they be destroyed at considerable cost.

Gowns

Indicated for use

- During aseptic procedures to protect the patient from infection.
- During non-aseptic procedures to protect staff members from possible contamination.
- Where the patient is susceptible to infection that may be transmitted via the staff member's body or clothes.

Instructions for use

- Reusable cotton gowns may be used to protect the wearer from casual or extensive contamination, e.g. when doing an aseptic or sterile procedure such as dressing extensive burn wounds. Cotton gowns are completely permeous and should be used only under controlled circumstances (e.g. in theatre as sterile gowns) and for specific patient-care procedures, such as wound-care. The gown is used once and discarded into the laundry, as it now has a significant bioburden of micro-organisms clinging to it. This makes using this type of gown very costly in terms of time and money, as enough gowns need to be available for isolation or other tasks. Cotton gowns must always be worn over or under plastic aprons so that the staff member's own clothing is protected from contamination that may soak into the material and dry on the gown, only to splinter or flake off later. Combining plastic aprons with cotton gowns also limits the transference of organisms from staff's bodies and their clothes to the patient. These gowns must be changed as soon as they become damp and not reused after drying – always launder the gowns before reusing.

- Sterilised cotton gowns only temporarily lower the count of micro-organisms in the susceptible patient's environment at the start of an aseptic procedure, e.g when caring for a small patient in a neonatal intensive-care unit. Once the gown has been exposed to air after removal from its packaging or has come into contact with the wearer's own clothes, it is no longer sterile.
- Special waterproof gowns are available for use in specific cases, e.g. during certain orthopaedic operations and when there is a high risk of contaminating healthcare staff with highly infectious matter (e.g. blood from haemorrhagic fever patients or extensive contamination with body fluid from a known infectious patient).
- Wash hands (or disinfect) before donning and after removing gowns to prevent any contamination of self or the environment.
- Store clean gowns where no accidental contamination is possible or unauthorised persons can handle them. Gowns that have to be reused should be hung singly so as not to contaminate the insides before reuse.

Eye protection/goggles/face shield

Indicated for use

- For personal protection of the eyes, oral and nasal mucosa and head against splatters of organic matter, chemical agents or careless contact of the face or head with soiled/contaminated hands.
- For protection of an immunosuppressed/ susceptible patients from infection origi-

nating from personnel's faces, airways or heads.

Instructions for use

- Avoid careless and unnecessary touching of the eye/face protector with contaminated hands.
- Wash or disinfect hands thoroughly before donning or removing the protector.
- Wash the protector with soap and water and dry it before reusing. Specialised protectors must be cleaned following the manufacturer's instructions.

Handling linen

Clean linen

Clean linen should be stored in a clean, dry area. Access to the linen store should be restricted to a few people only, to avoid casual contamination. Personnel must wash/disinfect their hands before handling clean linen.

Used, dry linen

Used, dry linen must be stripped from the bed, folded or rollled (singly) and then placed directly into laundry bags next to the patient's bedside. Used (soiled) linen should never be carried against the staff member's uniform as gross contamination leading to cross-infection occurs in this way. Environmental contamination soon follows. Staff members are also exposed to disease, although transmission to other susceptible patients is a greater risk.

Soiled/contaminated/wet linen

- Linen contaminated with or containing body fluids such as blood or any other unidentified fluid must be sealed in colour-coded plastic bags (e.g. yellow ones). Strip the bed and fold or roll the linen singly, then place in the plastic bags, which are then placed with (or in) the used, dry laundry bags. If the staff are aware of specific contagion that may be transmitted by the linen, biohazard stickers must be placed on the outside to warn laundry handlers and staff.

- Soiled or contaminated linen should never be sluiced in the patient-care area as this is environmentally contaminating. The same applies to disinfecting linen in a container in the patient-care area before transporting it to the laundry for washing.
- Contamination/soiling occurs readily in wet conditions and plastic bags encourage micro-organism proliferation because of the warm, damp atmosphere they generate.
- After soiled linen has been handled, personnel must wash/disinfect their hands before touching anything else.

Handling equipment/furniture

General guidelines

- Equipment and furniture should not be moved between infected, susceptible, or immune-compromised patients, especially those in protective isolation. As far as possible, patients in protective isolation should have separate equipment dedicated to their use. In unavoidable situations when equipment must be shared, strict control must be maintained to ensure that communal equipment is washed and/or disinfected according to the manufacturer's specifications/ward protocol to limit contamination before use by the next patient.
- Usually it is sufficient to wipe equipment with a paper towel soaked in an appropriate disinfectant, applying enough friction to remove micro-organisms from contaminated surfaces. If the item is visibly soiled, it should be washed with detergent and water if possible. Check the manufacturer's guide – ensure that items are compatible with the disinfectant/soap and water before applying them.

- Other measures used in infection control are pasteurisation, steam-autoclaving and gas sterilisation. An expert on the subject should, however, be consulted before any measure is used on a piece of equipment, to ensure that it is appropriate. Using incorrect methods of cleaning/disinfection may destroy costly equipment or expose patients or staff to harm.
- When equipment has been used in the care of patients with highly infectious or transmittable diseases, haemorrhaging, or when items are badly soiled, they should be 'double bagged' and identified with a biohazard sticker. If it is at all possible to rinse these items safely before sealing them in the bag, it should be done to protect the workers who have to handle and wash the equipment in the Pasteurisation or Central Sterilisation Services Department (CSSD) from contamination.
- Cutlery and crockery used by patients with highly contagious enteric or oral diseases or by extremely immune-compromised patients must be washed and stored separately from that caused by the other patients. Clean and dry cutlery and crockery carry few microbes until handled by staff.
- Whilst a patient is in isolation, all leftover food must be scraped into a plastic bag and discarded inside the room in a medical waste container before the plate is wiped with a paper towel. A basin with hot soapy water must be ready outside the patient's door and the used tableware dropped into it. This crockery and cutlery must be left until all the other patients' eating utensils have been washed. It can then be washed separately in fresh, hot soapy water, rinsed and air-dried.
- Disposable cutlery and crockery may be used for these patients (but may contribute to a feeling of alienation of the patient in isolation).
- Store crockery and cutlery where accidental

contamination is unlikely and unauthorised persons cannot soil the items.

- Bedpans and urinals should be removed as soon as possible after use. Only in cases of absolutely strict isolation should a used bedpan/urinal be left in the patient's room, in which case it must be covered with a clean cover. When these used bedpans and urinals are removed, the person must wear gloves, and be informed of the health hazard to him/herself. If a used urinal/bedpan has to be left in the patient's room, an appropriate liquid disinfectant must be poured over the contents. A 6-9 g sachet of dry chlorine-based disinfectant granules may be poured into a urinal with fluid contents, but the chlorine-based granules have to be dissolved in 100 ml of water before being used to cover solid contents of bedpans. Both containers must be emptied as soon as possible, rinsed with cold running water and washed/disinfected where appropriate.
- Careful hand hygiene before and after handling equipment is a prerequisite to prevent contamination of staff members, the patient or the environment.

Waste disposal

Clean, dry waste (household or non-infectious waste)

An appropriate coloured plastic bag (e.g. clear) can be used as a liner for the patients' waste bins so that refuse can be placed directly into them. Clean and dry paper, plastic and non-medical disposable items that have not had contact with the patient's body or body fluids are considered dry (non-medical) waste.

Small locker-bags at the bedside keep the bed and locker clean, and are handy for disposing of used facial tissues or other items.

Contaminated or soiled waste items

These are disposable items that have been in contact with or are contaminated by the body fluids/tissues of a patient. They are soiled/contaminated with organic matter, i.e. blood, wound drainage or mucous. Discarded used skin dressings, paper used for mopping up spillages of human origin, bloody swabs and any other disposable medical waste item must be discarded into refuse bins lined with a plastic bag the appropriate colour (e.g. red). When the bag is three quarters full it should be knotted in order to seal it before being removed for incineration. If the patient is suffering from a contagious disease, the plastic bag is double bagged, placed in a medical waste box, and identified with a biohazard sticker. Workers disposing of the refuse bags are then forewarned about the risk of contamination by hazardous microbes.

Staff and workers removing the waste should maintain proper hand hygiene before and after handling waste containers by specifically washing and/or disinfecting their hands with an antiseptic.

Liquid waste, e.g. vomitus, blood or aspirated body fluids

Liquid waste does not contain solids and can be poured down a sanitary sewer system, such as the sluice basin or a toilet bowl. The used container must be washed and disinfected or disposed of in a medical waste container.

Visitors

Visitors play a limited role in the spread of infection in healthcare facilities. Only the most general measures need mentioning:

- Visitors must be educated about proper hand hygiene in order to protect themselves, the patient and the environment from exposure to infection. The same principle applies to the use of protective clothing.
- Visitors need not use all the elaborate measures required from the nursing staff, as they tend to visit a single patient at a time. If they are going to visit more than one

person, the most infectious patient should be left till last. Staff, on the other hand, rotate from patient to patient whilst giving care and thus become the vehicle that spreads infection, therefore requiring more elaborate protective measures.

- Visitors should never be allowed to use the patients' toilets and other facilities, or to sit on the beds as they may bring contagion into the healthcare facility or carry it home with them as they leave.

Cleaning measures/environmental hygiene

General measures

- Cleaning staff must be supplied with the appropriate protective clothing/barriers in accordance with the risk that they run during their daily work. Gloves, impermeable aprons and boots must be supplied on an individual basis by the direct supervisor. It is also the supervisor's responsibility to see to it that the items are used correctly to prevent contamination/soiling of the person, patients or environment.
- Non-disposable cleaning equipment must be washed with detergent and water and dried before reuse. Washed items may also need additional pasteurisation or steam-autoclaving to render them totally contamination free, e.g. mop heads.
- Proper hand-washing/disinfection before and after cleaning procedures, as well as before meals is important for personal health among cleaning staff.
- Separate cleaning equipment must be provided for high-risk or possibly infectious areas such as toilets, ward laboratories,

sluices, and isolation rooms. These areas must be cleaned **after** the routine cleaning has been done in the rest of the department, so as to contain the possible spread of contamination/infection.

Additional measures

Patients in protective (reversed) isolation

- Staff must wear the necessary protective clothing and use the appropriate barriers to protect the **patient** against infection due to contamination/soiling originating from the environment, the staff or other patients.
- The patient's room must be cleaned **first**, before the rest of the ward/caregiving area.
- The professional staff are responsible for the work done by non-professionals and must ensure that they are trained and know what is expected from them.

Patients in source/direct isolation

The same principles apply as for protective isolation, except that the measures are now intended to protect the caregiver, i.e. the patient's room must be cleaned **last**, after the rest of the ward/caregiving area.

The summarised sheet that follows can be used in a patient-care area to list the basic infection prevention and control measures, which should be used to protect the patient, the staff and the environment. By marking the measures, the sheet can be included in each individual patient's file, for later auditing with the rest of the nursing documents. This relieves the staff of the trouble of rewriting all the measures each time there is an adjustment.

Basic infection prevention/control measures sheet

Name _____ Department _____ Date_____

The marked measures are indicated in the treatment of the above-mentioned patient/for protection of the hospital staff.

Measure	Motivation	Method
Hand-washing (compulsory)	Protects both the patient and the staff member against infection.	Wash soiled hands before and after each contact with warm water and ☐ antiseptic soap ☐ ordinary soap and dry thoroughly on a paper towel.
Hand disinfection (compulsory)	Protects the staff against contamination by transitory microbes that may cling to the skin. Protects the patient against contamination by these organisms.	Spray unsoiled hands with 5 ml of the disinfectant before and after each contact with the patient and/or his environment. Rub thoroughly over the whole hand and allow to air-dry spontaneously.
Room isolation	☐ Protective isolation for exposed patients ☐ Source isolation for suspected/confirmed infected patients.	Place in a single room with the door ☐ open ☐ closed.
Notification	Legally notifiable disease ☐ immediately (on suspicion) ☐ after laboratory confirmation.	Suspicion: contact the Infection Control Department. Other: the doctor/unit manager immediately completes and sends a GW 17/5 notice to the Infection Control Department.
Gloves	☐ For all contact with the patient ☐ For contact with body fluid/blood ☐ Protection of the susceptible patient ☐ For aseptic procedures.	☐ Unsterile gloves, worn once and then discarded ☐ Sterile gloves ☐ Available by the bedside.
☐ Plastic aprons ☐ Material gown	Protects the staff and the patient against contamination. ☐ For all contact with the patient ☐ For contact with body fluid/blood ☐ Protection of the susceptible patient ☐ For aseptic procedures.	Place inside the patient's room but hang singly to prevent contamination of the inside of the item. Gowns: single use each time. Aprons: mark the outside, reuse for 24 hours, wiping the outside with a paper towel and disinfectant each time.

Measure	Motivation	Method
Paper caps	Protect the staff and the patient against contamination ☐ For all contact with the patient ☐ For contact with body fluid/blood ☐ Protection of the susceptible patient ☐ For aseptic procedures.	Caps must cover all the hair. Single-use item. Use for a maximum of two hours at a time, or until the cap becomes damp or tears. Do not touch the cap unnecessarily.
Surgical face mask	Protects the staff and the patient against contamination. ☐ For all contact with the patient ☐ For contact with body fluid/blood ☐ Protection of the susceptible patient ☐ For aseptic procedures ☐ The patient may wear the mask.	Masks must cover the nose and mouth properly. All the ties must be fastened and the mask positioned under the chin. Single use item. Use for a maximum of two hours at a time, or until it becomes damp. Do not touch the mask unnecessarily.
Eye protection	Protects the staff members against splashes in the eyes. ☐ For all contact with the patient ☐ For exposure to splashes of body fluid/blood.	Preferably a personal-use item that must fit properly. Do not touch the item unnecessarily. Wash with soap and water after use and dry with a soft cloth to prevent scratching.
Visitors	Visiting this patient carries a risk of infection for the visitor.	Nursing staff remain responsible for the safety of anyone visiting the patient and must supervise the visit and use/discarding of protective clothing. Visitors may not use the patients' toilets or facilities. Visitors must visit healthier patients before seeing sicker/infective patients. ☐ Protective clothing needed ☐ Ensure that hands are washed before visitors leave the ward ☐ Restricted visiting ☐ No visitors allowed ☐ No children younger than 12 years allowed.

Measure	Motivation	Method
Equipment	This patient's contaminated equipment poses a risk of infection for other patients and staff members.	Do not move equipment around between patients. Equipment must be disinfected or washed in accordance with the instructions for use before shifting. Seal reusable equipment and instruments in clear plastic bags and send to CSSD for reprocessing.
Cleaning service	Cleaning this patient's environment poses a particular risk of infection for the cleaning staff.	Clean the room/environment ☐ first ☐ last. Use additional protective clothing: ☐ plastic aprons (single use) ☐ gloves (single use) ☐ face masks (single use).
Laundry	This patient's contaminated linen is a source of infection for other patients and staff members.	Seal all wet/infested linen in yellow plastic bags and send to the laundry. Mark severely soiled/infested linen as a warning measure.
Medical waste	This patient's medical waste is a greater source of infection to other patients, staff members, the community and the environment, than that of the rest of the hospital.	Seal all medical waste in red plastic bags, place in special containers after sealing. Seal the lid before removal to the storage area for incineration. ☐ Mark clearly as additional warning to all waste handlers.
Other measures	For protection of patients and staff members.	

Infection control officer _____ Date_____

2 Disease-specific infection prevention and control measures

ICD-10-B20 to B24	**ACQUIRED IMMUNODEFICIENCY SYNDROME** *(HTLV/LAV, HIV infection, AIDS, HIV)*

Signs and symptoms: A severe life-threatening condition, representing the late clinical stage of an infection that does progressive damage to the immune and other systems of the body (e.g. the nervous system). The level of immune incompetence determines the patient's prognosis and the course of the disease. The clinical symptoms vary between non-specific manifestations such as lymphadenopathy, anorexia, chronic diarrhoea, loss of weight, fever and prostration. Mouth and skin infections are usually the first signs that the patient's resistance is weakening. After activation, more specific symptoms develop: opportunistic infections (*Pneumocystis carinii* pneumonia, tuberculosis, chronic cryptosporidiosis, toxoplasmosis of the central nervous system, disseminated candidiasis, atypical mycobacteriosis, cytomegalovirus infection, herpes simplex infection, leukoencephalopathy) and cancers (Kaposi's sarcoma, primary B-cell lymphoma of the brain, and non-Hodgkin's lymphoma) are common. Additional indicator diseases include extrapulmonary tuberculosis, neurological manifestations such as dementia and sensory neuropathy, as well as wasting syndrome. Recurring septicaemia, pneumonia and reactivated pulmonary tuberculosis in a patient are indicators that further screening is needed to exclude the possibility of HIV infection. Some patients may be seroconverted but are clinically asymptomatic carriers. HIV-positive persons develop antibodies within 6–12 weeks although the period may be slightly longer under certain circumstances, e.g. after antiretroviral prophylaxis. As AIDS is a syndrome, any combination of symptoms may be present in a patient. Only detection of antibodies in the blood is an absolute indication of infection. The severity of HIV-related illnesses is dependent on the degree of immune system dysfunction.

Causative organism: A virus: human immunodeficiency virus (HIV).

Method of transmission: Contact with blood/sexual secretions of infected persons. Direct contact with body fluids or the tissues of an infected patient. Transfusion of infected blood products. Sharing of infected syringes and needles (drug users). Intrauterine/transplacental transmission. Injury with contaminated needles or other sharp objects. Transplantation of infected organs. Ingestion of infectious breast milk.

Incubation period:	Variable, possibly from shortly after infection until the death of patient. Approximately 50% of infected persons will have developed AIDS within 2–10 years after infection in the absence of antiretroviral treatment. The median incubation period in infants is shorter than in adults. Treatment lengthens the incubation period.
Infectious period:	From the time of infection, during the 'window period' and extends throughout the infected person's life. Communicability increases with increasing immune deficiency. Highest at seroconversion and just before death.

CONTROL/PREVENTATIVE MEASURES					
Barrier measures		**Protective clothing**		**Housekeeping**	
Hand washing	✓	Gloves	✓	Cleaning	R
Hand disinfection	✓	Masks	✓	Medical waste	R
Single room		Caps		Laundry	R
Private room + b/room		Eye protection			
Separate equipment		Cotton gowns			
Limit visitors		Plastic aprons			

Legal notification		**Readily communicable in the healthcare setting**	
On suspicion of infection		Yes	✓
On laboratory confirmation		No	

R = Routine   S = Special

Comments: In Africa, AIDS is predominantly a heterosexual disease. Intravenous drug users and all homosexual, bisexual and heterosexual persons with multiple sexual partners are especially at risk of contracting the disease. Tuberculosis and venereal diseases often occur in persons with AIDS. Infected persons must change their behaviour permanently; counselling and education on secondary control measures must commence as soon as possible after diagnosis of HIV. Healthcare staff should handle all sharp objects, as well as blood and blood products, with special care.

HIV-positive healthcare staff should stringently apply the standard precautions (detailed on page 171) when working with patients. This must be done to prevent the possible mutual transmission of opportunistic infecting pathogens from or to the staff member or patient. Infected staff members should not be placed in areas where they are routinely exposed to infected patients, such as medical, isolation or paediatric wards. In emergency units or operation theatres, these staff members should not work with cases where their hands are exposed to sharp bone shards or placed in body cavities where they cannot clearly see their fingers in relation to any sharp instruments being used. If it should happen that an infected staff member bleeds, or contaminates a patient with body fluid during a procedure, the patient and employer must be informed of the exposure. The same procedure in reverse must be followed as when a staff member has been exposed (refer to page 229). Staff members' CD4 count should be regularly monitored and any infections or AIDS-related secondary conditions treated immediately. When the HIV-positive person becomes too immunocompromised to work in safety, a decision regarding permanent or temporary suspension from work will need to be taken.

ICD-10-A22   ANTHRAX

Signs and symptoms:	An acute bacterial disease of the skin or lungs.
	Skin anthrax: Itching, skin lesions which become papular, then vesicular before developing a depressed black eschar. Untreated anthrax may spread to the lymph nodes and bloodstream, causing septicaemia.
	Respiratory anthrax: Initially mild, resembling any common upper respiratory infection, followed by acute respiratory distress, mediastinal widening, fever, shock, septicaemia and death.
Causative organism:	A bacillus: *Bacillus anthracis.*
Method of transmission:	Direct contact with or ingestion of skin/tissue of infected animals or the soil from the area where animals have died of anthrax. Inhalation of spores of the bacilli in dust. Person-to-person transmission with respiratory anthrax.
Incubation period:	2–7 days. Most cases within 48 hours.
Infectious period:	Soil or articles contaminated with spores may remain infective for many years.

CONTROL/PREVENTATIVE MEASURES

Barrier measures		Protective clothing		Housekeeping	
Hand washing	✓	Gloves	✓	Cleaning	S
Hand disinfection	✓	Masks	✓	Medical waste	R
Single room		Caps	✓	Laundry	R
Private room + b/room	✓	Eye protection	✓		
Separate equipment	✓	Cotton gowns	✓		
Limit visitors	✓	Plastic aprons	✓		

Legal notification		Readily communicable in the healthcare setting	
On suspicion of infection	✓	Yes	✓
On lab confirmation	✓	No	

R = Routine S = Special

Comments: Appropriate measures depend on the form of the disease. Steam sterilisation of all non-disposable contaminated/possibly contaminated articles should be used whenever possible to combat the spread of spores resistant to drying. Incineration of disposable items is safest. Contamination of the healthcare environment must be avoided at all costs! Airconditioning units must be switched off to prevent airborne dispersal of dust containing spores. This organism is often utilised as an airborne bioterrorism pathogen.

ICD-10-B77   ASCARIASIS *(Roundworm)*

Signs and symptoms:	An infestation of the small intestine that varies from asymptomatic to mild. Live worms passed orally, nasally or anally are often the first or only sign. **Pulmonary complaints:** Dyspnoea, irregular respiration, cough, fever and pneumonia. **Intestinal complaints:** Malabsorption of food, vomiting, abdominal pain, insomnia, obstruction and infestation of other digestive organs.
Causative organism:	A parasite: *Ascaris lumbricoides.*
Method of transmission:	Ingestion of raw contaminated food, water or soil (children). Not transmitted from person-to-person. Children between 3–8 years may reinfest themselves.
Incubation period:	Worms reach maturity within two months of ingestion of embryonic eggs.
Infectious period:	As long as an adult female worm in the intestine is capable of laying eggs. The normal life span is between 6–12 months during which +/-200 000 eggs are laid per day. The eggs may remain viable in soil for periods of months to years.

CONTROL/PREVENTATIVE MEASURES							
Barrier measures		**Protective clothing**		**Housekeeping**			
Hand washing	✓	Gloves	✓	Cleaning		R	
Hand disinfection	✓	Masks		Medical waste		R	
Single room		Caps		Laundry		R	
Private room + b/room		Eye protection					
Separate equipment		Cotton gowns					
Limit visitors		Plastic aprons					

Legal notification		**Readily communicable in the healthcare setting**		
On suspicion of infection		Yes		
On lab confirmation		No		✓

R = Routine   S = Special

Comments: Children and the mentally handicapped are the most susceptible to ascariasis. The worms are fairly large and resemble tapeworms. The eggs germinate in the intestine before migrating through the intestinal wall via the lymph- and bloodstreams to the liver and lungs where they develop further. The young adult larvae move up the bronchi to the pharynx where the infested person swallows them. The life cycle is completed when the adult female is fertilised in the intestine and lays her eggs before dying.

ICD-10-B44   ASPERGILLOSIS *(All species)*

Signs and symptoms:	A variety of non-specific symptoms are associated with aspergillosis. The fungus often affects the cornea, inner ear or lungs.
	Lung complications: Bronchial obstruction, nodule and abscess formation, empyema and pneumonia. In immune-compromised patients the infection may disseminate from the lungs to the brain, kidneys, and other organs, usually with fatal results. Various species of the genus produce aflatoxins.
Causative organism:	A fungus: *Aspergillus fumigatus* and *A. flavus* are the most common.
Method of transmission:	Inhalation of airborne spores that originate from the soil or environment, or from an infected person with an exuding lung abscess. Compost heaps and decaying or damp vegetation may harbour the fungi and facilitate spore production.
Incubation period:	Probably between days to weeks.
Infectious period:	As long as spores are present in the environment. Not transmitted from human to human.

CONTROL/PREVENTATIVE MEASURES

Barrier measures		Protective clothing		Housekeeping	
Hand washing	✓	Gloves	✓	Cleaning	R
Hand disinfection	✓	Masks	✓	Medical waste	R
Single room		Caps		Laundry	R
Private room + b/room	✓	Eye protection			
Separate equipment	✓	Cotton gowns			
Limit visitors	✓	Plastic aprons			

Legal notification		Readily communicable in the healthcare setting	
On suspicion of infection		Yes	
On lab confirmation		No	✓

R = Routine   S = Special

Comments: The greatest risk is the contamination of the environment of the immune-compromised or mechanically ventilated patient as well as that of patients receiving cytotoxic/chemotherapy treatment. Healthy persons are not at risk of contracting the disease, but may act as vehicles of transmission to susceptible patients.

ICD-10-J11.0 -J11.1   AVIAN INFLUENZA A *(Highly pathogenic avian influenza, HPAI, avian flu, fowl plague, bird flu)*

Signs and symptoms:	An acute respiratory illness characterised by fever higher than 38°C, cough, conjunctivitis, sore throat, fatigue, respiratory difficulty and severe, often fulminant pneumonia.
Causative organism:	An influenza virus – HPAI, subtype H5N1, usually carried by asymptomatic waterfowl, who excrete large volumes of viral particles in their faeces.
Method of transmission:	Usually only infects birds and sometimes pigs. Not normally spread to humans, but some cases have been reported as a direct result of contact with infected live and dead birds, their droppings (inhaling aerosolised faeces) and respiratory secretions.
Incubation period:	Average 10 days.
Infectious period:	Historically most people who become infected are immune to re-infection. Birds that survive excrete the virus for at least 10 days in oral secretions and droppings.

CONTROL/PREVENTATIVE MEASURES

Barrier measures		Protective clothing		Housekeeping	
Hand washing	✓	Gloves	✓	Cleaning	R
Hand disinfection	✓	Masks: N95 high-particulate filter type	✓	Medical waste	R
Single room		Caps	✓	Laundry	R
Private room + b/room	✓	Eye protection	✓		
Separate equipment	✓	Cotton gowns			
Limit visitors	✓	Plastic aprons	✓		

Legal notification		Readily communicable in the healthcare setting	
On suspicion of infection		Yes	
On lab confirmation		No	✓

R = Routine   S = Special

Comments: No specific vaccine is available at present, though it has been recommended that poultry handlers should be vaccinated with current human influenza vaccine to diminish the possibility of dual infection, and should routinely wear high particulate filter masks at work. Any healthcare workers exposed to the secretions of infected patients are at risk of contracting HPAI. The virus is deactivated by 70% alcohol and sodium hypochlorite. Reports of a growing number of countries, including South Africa, isolating highly virulent avian influenza viruses in poultry is of particular concern to the World Health Organization. Because influenza viruses are unstable and prone to genetic mutation, and H5N1 especially so, the fear exists that a new influenza virus subtype may develop which can jump species, in situations where high viral loads are present in one species. Humans could be susceptible, as they would have had no previous contact with the new virus strain. The World Health Organization has activated an influenza pandemic plan, and traveller's warnings are issued as needed. When travelling to an area where there have been reports of HVAI outbreaks, tourists should avoid visiting areas soiled with animal blood and secretions, any contact with live poultry and their droppings, uncooked chicken and raw eggs. The virus may be present in droppings on soiled eggshells. Careful and frequent hand hygiene (washing, or disinfection with a waterless alcohol-based rub) is essential. Care should be taken that only cooked, hygienically prepared food is eaten, as the virus is destroyed by heat.

ICD-10-B65.9   BILHARZIA *(Bilharziasis, schistosomiasis)*

Signs and symptoms:	A blood fluke infection where adult male and female worms live out a life span lasting several years in the host's mesenteric and/or vesicle veins. Symptoms include diarrhoea, abdominal pain, an enlarged liver and spleen, haematuria and dysuria, liver fibrosis, portal hypertension, central nervous abnormalities and general cystitis.
Causative organism:	A blood trematode: *Schistosoma mansoni*, *S. haematobium* and *S. japonicum* are the most common species.
Method of transmission:	Ingestion of water containing larvae of the flukes or the urine/excreta of infected persons while swimming, walking or working in contaminated water. The larvae penetrate the skin, then migrate via the bloodstream to the liver, lungs and abdomen.
Incubation period:	Acute systemic symptoms (Katayama fever) may occur in primary infections at the time that worms reach maturity and start depositing eggs – usually 2–6 weeks after infection.
Infectious period:	No direct person-to-person transfer but infected persons may spread the infestation by discharging eggs in their urine or faeces for 5-10 years or longer. Infected snails may release larvae for periods of weeks up to months.

CONTROL/PREVENTATIVE MEASURES						
Barrier measures		**Protective clothing**		**Housekeeping**		
Hand washing	✓	Gloves	✓	Cleaning		R
Hand disinfection	✓	Masks		Medical waste		R
Single room		Caps		Laundry		R
Private room + b/room		Eye protection				
Separate equipment		Cotton gowns				
Limit visitors		Plastic aprons				

Legal notification		**Readily communicable in the healthcare setting**		
On suspicion of infection		Yes		
On lab confirmation		No		✓

R = Routine   S = Special

Comments: In endemic areas the population should be informed about preventative measures and personal hygiene. Where exposure to contaminated water is suspected, the skin should be dried thoroughly and 70% alcohol applied to destroy surface cercariae (larvae). Supervised medical treatment is important to the future health of the patient. Water can be treated with chlorine or iodine, and allowed to stand for 48–72 hours before use in the home.

ICD-10-A23   BRUCELLOSIS *(Malta fever)*

Signs and symptoms:	An acute or insidious onset with a fluctuating fever, profuse sweating, rigor, weakness, headache, depression, loss of weight, and generalised muscle pain. The disease may last between days and months.
Causative organism:	A bacterium: *Brucella abortus.*
Method of transmission:	Direct contact with the tissue, secretions, milk and placentas of infected animals/cattle. Airborne transfer amongst animals is common.
Incubation period:	5–60 days, with an average of 30 days.
Infectious period:	Apparently no person-to-person transfer.

CONTROL/PREVENTATIVE MEASURES

Barrier measures		Protective clothing		Housekeeping	
Hand washing	✓	Gloves	✓	Cleaning	R
Hand disinfection	✓	Masks		Medical waste	R
Single room		Caps	✓	Laundry	R
Private room + b/room		Eye protection	✓		
Separate equipment		Cotton gowns	✓		
Limit visitors		Plastic aprons	✓		

Legal notification		Readily communicable in the healthcare setting	
On suspicion of infection		Yes	
On lab confirmation	✓	No	✓

R = Routine   S = Special

Comments: Pasteurisation of the milk from all cows, goats and sheep is necessary. Infected animals are usually destroyed. A certificate of good health has to be produced before a farmer whose stock has been infected may sell dairy products commercially. Relapse of the disease may occur in about 15% of treated cases.

ICD-10-B37   CANDIDIASIS *(Thrush, moniliasis)*

Signs and symptoms:	A mycosis, usually of the mouth or other mucous membranes such as the gastrointestinal tract, bladder or vagina. Common in small babies, immune-compromised patients (e.g. HIV-positive, diabetic, cancer or mechanically ventilated patients) and persons using broad-spectrum antibiotics.
Causative organism:	A fungus: most commonly *Candida albicans, C. tropicalis, C. torulopsis* and *C. glabrata*.
Method of transmission:	Contact with the secretions of the mouth, mucous membranes or skin of infected patients; during childbirth from mother to neonate.
Incubation period:	2–5 days.
Infectious period:	As long as the viable pathogen is present in blood or tissues, other than its normal habitat.

CONTROL/PREVENTATIVE MEASURES

Barrier measures		Protective clothing		Housekeeping	
Hand washing	✓	Gloves	✓	Cleaning	R
Hand disinfection	✓	Masks		Medical waste	R
Single room		Caps		Laundry	R
Private room + b/room		Eye protection			
Separate equipment	✓	Cotton gowns			
Limit visitors		Plastic aprons	✓		

Legal notification		Readily communicable in the healthcare setting	
On suspicion of infection		Yes	
On lab confirmation		No	✓

R = Routine   S = Special

Comments: In the Maternity Department, infected babies are isolated in incubators or kept with their mothers. Keep feeding bottles, teats, and pacifiers separate, then wash and boil after use. Disseminated candidiasis may cause lesions of the brain, kidneys, lungs, liver and spleen. Cardiac valve prostheses as well as any implantable temporary or permanent intravascular devices are prone to contamination following infection with candida. In a normally healthy person, confirmed laboratory cultures showing candidiasis may indicate the presence of a latent immune-compromising disease like HIV or auto-immune suppression, and should be investigated further.

ICD-10-A57 **CHANCROID** *(Ulcus molle, soft chancre)*

Signs and symptoms:	An acute localised infection characterised by single or multiple painful necrotising ulcers at the inoculation site. Swelling or suppuration of the surrounding lymph nodes commonly occurs. The infection may present asymptomatically or mild symptoms (that pass unnoticed because of the hidden ulcer on the cervical or vaginal mucosa) may occur.
Causative organism:	A bacterium: *Haemophilus ducreyi* (Ducrey bacillus).
Method of transmission:	Sexually transmitted, or through direct contact with the secretions of open lesions or pus from suppurating lymph nodes.
Incubation period:	3–5 days; maximum 14 days.
Infectious period:	As long as the organisms are present in the primary lesion or pus from suppurating lymph nodes. It may take weeks for all the lesions to heal. Auto-infection of other skin areas is possible if the personal hygiene of the infected person is poor.

CONTROL/PREVENTATIVE MEASURES

Barrier measures		Protective clothing		Housekeeping	
Hand washing	✓	Gloves	✓	Cleaning	R
Hand disinfection	✓	Masks		Medical waste	R
Single room		Caps		Laundry	R
Private room + b/room		Eye protection			
Separate equipment	✓	Cotton gowns			
Limit visitors		Plastic aprons	✓		

Legal notification		Readily communicable in the healthcare setting	
On suspicion of infection		Yes	
On lab confirmation		No	✓

R = Routine   S = Special

Comments: Avoid sexual contact until the treatment has been completed (2–3 weeks). Education on personal hygiene is necessary to combat spread of the infection. Sexual partners have to be treated as well.

Genital ulcers are strongly associated with an increased risk of HIV infection. Sexual promiscuity and poor personal hygiene promotes the spread of the infection. Women may unknowingly be carriers of the infection as they may present without any visible signs and symptoms.

ICD-10-B01   CHICKENPOX *(Varicella)*

Signs and symptoms:	A highly communicable viral disease that usually affects children. An acute onset with slight fever and a skin eruption which is maculopapular for a few hours and vesicular for 3–4 days, developing a granular scab. Lesions commonly occur in different stages of maturity and are more abundant on the covered areas of the body. Mild, atypical and unapparent infections occur. The symptoms are more severe in adults than in children.
Causative organism:	A virus: the varicella zoster virus (a herpes virus).
Method of transmission:	Direct contact with the vesicle fluid, droplets or airborne spread of secretions from the respiratory tract. Indirect transfer through infected objects, e.g. toys.
Incubation period:	13–21 days, usually about 17 days.
Infectious period:	2–5 days before onset of the rash until six days after appearance of the first vesicles. Immunocompromised or immunised persons may remain infectious for a longer time.

CONTROL/PREVENTATIVE MEASURES					
Barrier measures		**Protective clothing**		**Housekeeping**	
Hand washing	✓	Gloves	✓	Cleaning	S
Hand disinfection	✓	Masks	✓	Medical waste	R
Single room	✓	Caps		Laundry	R
Private room + b/room		Eye protection			
Separate equipment	✓	Cotton gowns			
Limit visitors	✓	Plastic aprons	✓		

Legal notification		**Readily communicable in the healthcare setting**	
On suspicion of infection		Yes	✓
On lab confirmation		No	

R = Routine   S = Special

Comments: Immunisation is available for children and adults. Allow immune healthcare workers to care for infectious patients. Infection during the first trimester of pregnancy may cause congenital abnormalities in the foetus. Good hand hygiene is important because of the extreme contagiousness of varicella. Adult patients are more severely afflicted by the infection than children. By the time the rash appears, the child usually feels better. Patients may return to school or work as soon as they are free of vesicles or scabs. The same virus causes shingles.

ICD-10-A00   CHOLERA

Signs and symptoms:	An acute intestinal disease with sudden onset, profuse watery stools, a normal temperature and occasional vomiting. Rapid dehydration, acidosis and circulatory collapse may cause death within a few hours. Stools may contain blood and large volumes of mucus. Mostly the infection is mild and may even be asymptomatic.
Causative organism:	A bacterium: *Vibrio cholerae* (especially the *El Tor* biotype).
Method of transmission:	Ingestion of contaminated food or water.
Incubation period:	From a few hours to 5 days, average usually 2–3 days.
Infectious period:	As long as the organism is present in the stools, up to one week after the last episode of diarrhoea. The carrier stage may persist for months. Normally most well-fed adults are not (overly) susceptible to the disease.

CONTROL/PREVENTATIVE MEASURES

Barrier measures		Protective clothing		Housekeeping	
Hand washing	✓	Gloves	✓	Cleaning	R
Hand disinfection	✓	Masks		Medical waste	R
Single room		Caps		Laundry	R
Private room + b/room	✓	Eye protection			
Separate equipment	✓	Cotton gowns			
Limit visitors		Plastic aprons	✓		

Legal notification		Readily communicable in the healthcare setting	
On suspicion of infection		Yes	
On lab confirmation	✓	No	✓

R = Routine   S = Special

Comments: Disinfection/sterilisation of articles that have come into contact with the secretions (vomitus or stool) of cholera patients is recommended, after washing with soap and warm water. Rehydration of toddlers and babies is vital as diarrhoea and vomiting causes rapid dehydration that can lead to circulatory collapse and death. Exclusion from school and work is indicated for 7 days after the last diarrhoeal episode. Contacts of patients must be followed up and investigated. Early rehydration and electrolyte replacement is necessary, especially in children (5 ml table salt, 5 ml bicarbonate of soda, and 20 ml sugar, dissolved in 1 litre of boiled, cooled water may be used as an oral rehydration solution).

ICD-10-J00   COMMON COLD *(Coryza, acute viral rhinitis, acute nasopharyngitis)*

Signs and symptoms:	An acute catarrhal infection of the upper respiratory tract; characterised by sneezing, coryza, lacrimation, irritated nasopharynx, chills and malaise. Usually lasts 2–7 days. High fever is common in children younger than +/-3 years but is rare in adults. Laryngitis, tracheitis or bronchitis may occur. Sinusitis and otitis media may be general complications of the common cold.
Causative organism:	Viruses: Rhinovirus (of which there are more than 100 known serotypes) corona-, para-, influenza, adeno- and entero- viruses are but a few common examples.
Method of transmission:	Presumably through direct contact or inhalation of droplets in the air; indirectly through contact with hands or other fomites freshly soiled with nasal and throat discharges from an infected person.
Incubation period:	Usually 12–72 hours, on average 48 hours.
Infectious period:	Presumably from 24 hours before the onset of symptoms until 5 days after.

CONTROL/PREVENTATIVE MEASURES						
Barrier measures		**Protective clothing**		**Housekeeping**	
Hand washing	✓	Gloves	✓	Cleaning	R
Hand disinfection	✓	Masks		Medical waste	R
Single room		Caps		Laundry	R
Private room + b/room		Eye protection			
Separate equipment		Cotton gowns			
Limit visitors		Plastic aprons			

Legal notification		**Readily communicable in the healthcare setting**	
On suspicion of infection		Yes	✓
On lab confirmation		No	

R = Routine   S = Special

Comments: The common cold affects concentration and work performance. The average person develops 1–6 colds a year. The incidence is highest in children younger than 5 years and decreases with age. Contaminated hands readily transfer the virus to the mucosa of the nose or eyes. Overcrowding encourages the spread of the infection. Vaccination is available against some of the viruses. Susceptible persons should avoid sick persons. Work/school exclusion is unnecessary. The most important point to remember is that good hand hygiene will protect most persons from accidental transfer through contact.

ICD-10-B30   CONJUNCTIVITIS *(Pinkeye)*

Signs and symptoms:	Increased lachrymation, redness (hyperaemia), pain or irritation (itchiness), oedema of the eyelids, photophobia, mucopurulent discharge of one or both eyes. Haemorrhages may follow an extended virus infection. Corneal ulceration is rare.
Causative organism:	**Bacterial:** Most commonly due to *Haemophilus influenzae (H. aegyptius)* or *Streptococcus pneumoniae.* **Viral:** Mostly a picornavirus or adenovirus.
Method of transmission:	Contact with the eye and/or nasal secretions of infected persons as well as contaminated clothing, towels, cosmetics, hands, eye makeup or multi-dose eyedrop containers. Reinfection of an individual is common if good hand and personal hygiene is not promoted or where people live in close proximity to each other.
Incubation period:	24–72 hours for bacterial infection. Viral infections vary.
Infectious period:	As long as viable bacteria is found in the eye secretions, usually 2 days to a maximum 2–3 weeks. Virus infections usually last 4–6 days and remain contagious for 4–14 days after the first symptoms appear.

CONTROL/PREVENTATIVE MEASURES

Barrier measures		Protective clothing		Housekeeping	
Hand washing	✓	Gloves	✓	Cleaning	R
Hand disinfection	✓	Masks		Medical waste	R
Single room		Caps		Laundry	R
Private room + b/room		Eye protection			
Separate equipment	✓	Cotton gowns			
Limit visitors		Plastic aprons	✓		

Legal notification		Readily communicable in the healthcare setting	
On suspicion of infection		Yes, in paediatric wards	✓
On lab confirmation		No	

R = Routine   S = Special

Comments: A highly contagious disease, especially amongst children. Good hand and personal hygiene is essential to combat the infection. School/work exclusion is important until the eyes are clear and no more exudates or redness are apparent. The elderly as well as children younger than 5 years are especially prone to pinkeye whilst the middle-aged group is usually more immune. Contaminated clothing and towels may transmit the infection among household contacts. Dust, cold and wind aggravate the condition.

ICD-10-B25 CYTOMEGALOVIRUS INFECTIONS

Signs and symptoms:	**Perinatal:** Lethargy, convulsions, jaundice, subcutaneous haemorrhage, microcephaly, mental retardation, motor disability, loss of hearing, chronic liver disease, coma and death in severely afflicted babies. These neonates have a high mortality rate. Infection later in life has less impact on a patient, except if a pregnant woman is infected or the condition flares up again (reactivation).
Causative organism:	A virus: the cytomegalovirus (a human herpes virus).
Method of transmission:	Direct contact with tissues, blood or the secretions of an infected person. The virus is present in breast milk, urine, saliva and sexual discharges. Intrauterine infection, as well as infection after organ or tissue transplants may occur.
Incubation period:	Difficult to determine. Infection may occur in the uterus, during delivery or shortly afterwards. Contagion follows within 3–12 weeks after delivery and 3–8 weeks after transplant or transfusion with contaminated blood. Susceptible adults may be infected through contact with infected children's urine.
Infectious period:	May last months or even years. May recur again during pregnancy or periods of temporary immune suppression in healthy persons. After neonatal infection, a child may shed the virus for the first 5–6 years. Most adults are not susceptible to infection.

CONTROL/PREVENTATIVE MEASURES					
Barrier measures		**Protective clothing**		**Housekeeping**	
Hand washing	✓	Gloves	✓	Cleaning	R
Hand disinfection	✓	Masks		Medical waste	R
Single room		Caps		Laundry	R
Private room + b/room		Eye protection			
Separate equipment	✓	Cotton gowns			
Limit visitors	✓	Plastic aprons	✓		

Legal notification		Readily communicable in the healthcare setting	
On suspicion of infection		Yes	
On lab confirmation		No	✓

R = Routine   S = Special

Comments: Less than 3% of all healthy adults are asymptomatic pharyngeal carriers of the virus, which they unknowingly spread. Proper hand hygiene and good housekeeping by all staff members should be maintained at all times. Immunosuppressed patients, the newborn and all pregnant workers from the maternity or paediatric wards, as well as organ transplant patients are at risk of infection inside as well as outside the hospital. Infection with the cytomegalovirus seldom produces severe symptomatic disease and is usually very mild or asymptomatic from shortly after birth. If the infection does occur later, the clinical symptoms usually depend on the age and immune status of the patient.

ICD-10-A36   DIPHTHERIA

Signs and symptoms:	An acute infection of the throat, tonsils, pharynx, larynx, and nose and the surrounding skin and mucous membranes. Patches of greyish pseudo - membrane surrounded by a red inflammatory area mark the characteristic lesion, caused by the secretion of a specific cytotoxin. Lymph nodes are enlarged, tender and swollen. The throat is sore. Extreme swelling of the lymph nodes and/or tissues (oedema) may be present (causing the 'bull neck' appearance). Fever may be mild to high. In severe cases of laryngeal diphtheria respiratory obstruction is caused when the pseudo-membrane closes off the airway. This may be fatal, especially in babies and young children. Nasal diphtheria is mostly mild and may present only as a chronic 'runny nose'.
Causative organism:	A bacterium: *Corynebacterium diphtheriae.*
Method of transmission:	Commonly spread through droplets (even during speech), ingestion of unpasteurised contaminated milk or contact with contaminated fomites such as handkerchiefs or hands.
Incubation period:	2–5 days, sometimes as long as 10 days.
Infectious period:	2–4 weeks, or till no more viable bacilli are present in the nasopharynx. Untreated carriers may (unwittingly) spread the infection for periods up to 6 months or longer. Effective antibiotic treatment contains infectiveness within 24–48 hours.

CONTROL/PREVENTATIVE MEASURES

Barrier measures		Protective clothing		Housekeeping	
Hand washing	✓	Gloves	✓	Cleaning	S
Hand disinfection	✓	Masks	✓	Medical waste	R
Single room		Caps		Laundry	R
Private room + b/room	✓	Eye protection			
Separate equipment	✓	Cotton gowns			
Limit visitors	✓	Plastic aprons	✓		

Legal notification		Readily communicable in the healthcare setting	
On suspicion of infection		Yes	
On lab confirmation	✓	No	✓

R = Routine   S = Special

Comments: Recovery from the clinical infection is not always followed by lifelong immunity. Passive immunisation is no guarantee of immunity either. The passive immunity with which babies are born is lost before the sixth month. Antitoxin only supplies temporary immunity (+/-15–21 days) while toxoid provides a longer period but has more side-effects. A programme of immunisation has to be completed following a set schedule (4 doses). All intimate (household) or close contacts of the patient must be monitored for 7 days to identify any symptoms.

Nasal carriers must be identified and treated. Nasal and throat swabs should only be taken 24–48 hours after the last antibiotic was administered. If laboratory facilities are not available to verify the diagnosis, the infected person must be isolated from other patients for at least 14 days after commencing treatment on suspicion of the diagnosis. Recuperated healthcare staff, food handlers and child minders should submit nose and throat swabs before returning to work. Exclusion from work and school should be maintained until 2 consecutive nose and throat swabs are cultured negative.

ICD-10-A 98.3   EBOLA *(Ebola fever, Ebola viral haemorrhagic fever)*

Signs and symptoms:	Acute, sudden onset characterised by fever, headache, myalgia, pharyngitis, malaise. Weakness, followed by diarrhoea, vomiting and abdominal pain, hepatic damage, renal failure, terminal shock and multi-organ failure. Some patients develop a maculopapular skin rash, bloodshot eyes, hiccups, and internal and external bleeding.
Causative organism:	Ebola virus: Ebola HF.
Method of transmission:	An African zoonosis (animal-borne infection) of which the natural reservoir (origin, locations and habitat) is as yet unknown. Nosocomial person-to-person transmission due to direct contact with infected blood, secretions, organs or semen is possible.
Incubation period:	2–21 days.
Infectious period:	As long as viable virus is present in blood and secretions. Transmission through semen has occurred up to 7 weeks after clinical recovery.

CONTROL/PREVENTATIVE MEASURES

Barrier measures		Protective clothing		Housekeeping	
Hand washing	✓	Gloves	✓	Cleaning	S
Hand disinfection	✓	Masks	✓	Medical waste	S
Single room		Caps	✓	Laundry	S
Private room + b/room	✓	Eye protection	✓		
Separate equipment	✓	Impermeable gowns	✓		
Limit visitors	✓	Plastic aprons			

Legal notification		Readily communicable in the healthcare setting	
On suspicion of infection	✓	Yes	✓
On lab confirmation	✓	No	

R = Routine   S = Special

Comments: There is no standard treatment for Ebola. Patients receive supportive treatment – balancing fluids and electrolytes, maintaining tissue and pulmonary oxygenation, maintaining blood circulation by replacing blood loss, and treating complications symptomatically. Sexual intercourse should be restricted for 3 months after recovery or until semen is shown to be free of the virus.

ICD-10-A83 to A86   ENCEPHALITIS

Signs and symptoms:	A group of acute inflammatory diseases that differ from mild to severe affliction of the brain, meninges and spinal cord. Often the infection presents asymptomatically with headache as the most severe complaint. More severe affliction usually presents with an acute onset, severe headache, pyrexia, nausea, vomiting, disorientation, stupor, coma, spasticity, tremors, convulsions, drowsiness and/or paralysis. In very severe cases epilepsy has been noted, especially where tick-borne spread is suspected. Neurological lesions may be permanent, depending on the age of the patient and the infective organism. Encephalitis is often one of the complications of more common infectious diseases such as measles, rubella, chickenpox, herpes simplex or zoster, syphilis, tuberculosis and poliomyelitis. Some types of vaccine may also cause mild symptoms of encephalitis.
Causative organism:	Different species of virus or bacteria.
Method of transmission:	The bite of an infected mosquito, flea or tick (depending on the type of infection) or the migration of organisms from a primary focus of infection.
Incubation period:	5–15 days.
Infectious period :	Not transmittable from person-to-person. Mosquitoes and ticks remain infective lifelong. In the human host the viraemia lasts for 7–10 days. Infection leads to active immunity against the specific causative organism. Children are particularly susceptible to the infection via another contagious condition such as chickenpox.

CONTROL/PREVENTATIVE MEASURES

Barrier measures		Protective clothing		Housekeeping	
Hand washing	✓	Gloves	✓	Cleaning	R
Hand disinfection	✓	Masks		Medical waste	R
Single room		Caps		Laundry	R
Private room + b/room		Eye protection			
Separate equipment		Cotton gowns			
Limit visitors		Plastic aprons	✓		

Legal notification		Readily communicable in the healthcare setting	
On suspicion of infection		Yes	
On lab confirmation		No	✓

R = Routine S = Special

Comments: Viral encephalitis is usually not contagious. The patients usually complain of a severe headache, and this is the reason most are accommodated singly. Where necessary, infection control measures are taken in accordance with the primary causative condition, e.g. the use of insect repellents in the environment as well as symptomatic treatment/support of the individual patient.

ICD-10-A05 FOOD POISONING: BOTULISM

Signs and symptoms:	A severe intoxication (not an infection). Primary nerve involvement: double vision, dry mouth, sore throat, vomiting and diarrhoea (sometimes constipation). Symmetrical descending flaccid paralysis may follow these symptoms. About one third of patients die within 3–7 days after the onset, usually from respiratory failure or superimposed infections. Fever is absent.
Causative organism:	Toxins produced by the bacterium *Clostridium botulinum*. Boiling destroys the toxin. Ordinary refrigeration of 4°C or lower does not destroy the spores.
Method of transmission:	Ingestion of food containing the toxin. Possible sources are raw or smoked meat, inadequately heated canned products, fish and seafood. Wound infection may lead to secondary botulism as well.
Incubation period:	Usually 12–36 hours after eating contaminated food, sometimes several days later. Generally, the shorter the period, the more severe the disease and the higher the fatality rate.
Infectious period:	None. The symptoms are caused by toxins and not micro-organisms.

CONTROL/PREVENTATIVE MEASURES						
Barrier measures		**Protective clothing**		**Housekeeping**	
Hand washing	✓	Gloves	✓	Cleaning		R
Hand disinfection	✓	Masks		Medical waste		R
Single room		Caps		Laundry		R
Private room + b/room		Eye protection				
Separate equipment	✓	Cotton gowns				
Limit visitors	✓	Plastic aprons				

Legal notification		Readily communicable in the healthcare setting	
On suspicion of infection		Yes/No	Yes
On lab confirmation. Only if four or more cases have been diagnosed from the same food source			✓

R = Routine S = Special

Comments: Incinerate contaminated food, and steam autoclave all equipment. Mechanical patient ventilation may be necessary. Notification of the local authority is compulsory by law when more than four persons have acquired the food poisoning from the same source. In neonates or newborn babies botulism may develop into necrotic enteritis, which may be fatal.

ICD-10-A05.2   FOOD POISONING: CLOSTRIDIUM

Signs and symptoms:	A severe intoxication (not an infection). Sudden onset of colic followed by diarrhoea, nausea is common but fever and vomiting are usually absent. A mild disease of short duration. Seldom fatal in healthy persons.
Causative organism:	The enterotoxin of bacteria: type A strains of *Clostridium perfringens (C. welchii)* cause typical food poisoning symptoms; type C strains have caused necrotising enteritis. Heat-resistant spores germinate and multiply during lengthy cooling and reheating of food.
Method of transmission:	Ingestion of food contaminated with soil or faeces (especially food and meat not properly cooked or reheated). Large numbers of organisms are required to produce clinical symptoms.
Incubation period:	6–24 hours, usually 10–12 hours.
Infectious period:	None. The symptoms are caused by toxins and not micro-organisms.

CONTROL/PREVENTATIVE MEASURES						
Barrier measures		**Protective clothing**		**Housekeeping**		
Hand washing	✓	Gloves	✓	Cleaning		R
Hand disinfection	✓	Masks		Medical waste		R
Single room		Caps		Laundry		R
Private room + b/room		Eye protection				
Separate equipment	✓	Cotton gowns				
Limit visitors		Plastic aprons	✓			

Legal notification		Readily communicable in the healthcare setting	
On suspicion of infection		Yes/No	No
On lab confirmation. Only if four or more cases have been diagnosed from the same food source			✓

R = Routine   S = Special

Comments: Notification of the local authority is compulsory when four or more patients have acquired the poisoning from the same source. Adults seldom need hospitalisation, except when complications arise.

ICD-10-A05   FOOD POISONING: STAPHYLOCOCCAL

Signs and symptoms:	An intoxication (not an infection) with an abrupt onset, severe nausea, vomiting and abdominal cramps, usually diarrhoea, prostration as well as a low to subnormal temperature. Haematemesis may occur with severe vomiting.
Causative organism:	The toxin of the bacteria *Staphylococcus aureus* (a heat-resistant enterotoxin).
Method of transmission:	Ingestion of food containing the toxin. The contamination may originate from infected persons or animals – an infected person may contaminate food while handling it with unwashed hands, causing the toxin-producing staphylococci to multiply in the food.
Incubation period:	30 minutes to 6 hours, usually 2–4 hours from the time of ingestion until the first symptoms appear.
Infectious period:	None. The symptoms are caused by toxins and not micro-organisms.

CONTROL/PREVENTATIVE MEASURES							
Barrier measures		**Protective clothing**		**Housekeeping**		
Hand washing	✓	Gloves	✓	Cleaning		R
Hand disinfection	✓	Masks		Medical waste		R
Single room		Caps		Laundry		R
Private room + b/room		Eye protection				
Separate equipment	✓	Cotton gowns				
Limit visitors		Plastic aprons	✓			

Legal notification		**Readily communicable in the healthcare setting**	
On suspicion of infection		Yes/No	No
On lab confirmation. Only if four or more cases have been diagnosed from the same food source			✓

R = Routine   S = Special

Comments: Notification to the local authority is compulsory when four or more persons acquire the disease from the same food source.

ICD-A08.0   GASTRO-ENTERITIS: ROTAVIRUS

Signs and symptoms:	A sporadic severe infection with watery diarrhoea, fever and vomiting that may lead to (fatal) dehydration. At times the infection presents sub-clinically. Common in babies and young children. Spreads readily in hospitals and care facilities. On average the symptoms usually last for 4–6 days.
Causative organism:	A virus: rotavirus, especially Group A.
Method of transmission:	Probably faecal-oral but may possibly be faecal-respiratory as well. Contact transmission is possible.
Incubation period:	Approximately 24–72 hours, on average 48 hours.
Infectious period:	During the acute stage, up to +/-8 days after the appearance of the first symptoms.

CONTROL/PREVENTATIVE MEASURES

Barrier measures		Protective clothing		Housekeeping	
Hand washing	✓	Gloves	✓	Cleaning	R
Hand disinfection	✓	Masks		Medical waste	R
Single room		Caps		Laundry	R
Private room + b/room	✓	Eye protection			
Separate equipment	✓	Cotton gowns			
Limit visitors	✓	Plastic aprons	✓		

Legal notification		Readily communicable in the healthcare setting	
On suspicion of infection		Yes	✓
On lab confirmation		No	

R = Routine S = Special

Comments: Susceptibility is highest amongst children aged 6–24 months. Most children are infected during their first four years of life. By the age of 3, most children have developed anti-bodies against the rotavirus strains. The infection is most prevalent during the colder winter months. Good personal hygiene has to be maintained at all times. Infected infants less than 3 months of age do not commonly present with diarrhoea.

ICD-10 A08.1   GASTRO-ENTERITIS: VIRAL

Signs and symptoms:	Nausea, vomiting, diarrhoea, abdominal- and muscle pain, dehydration, headache, mild fever and exhaustion. Symptoms are self-limiting and usually last 24–48 hours.
Causative organism:	Different viruses, excluding rotavirus.
Method of transmission:	Probably faecal-oral. Possibly through the ingestion of contaminated food or water.
Incubation period:	24–48 hours.
Infectious period:	During the acute phase of the infection until shortly thereafter.

CONTROL/PREVENTATIVE MEASURES						
Barrier measures		Protective clothing		Housekeeping	
Hand washing	✓	Gloves	✓	Cleaning	R
Hand disinfection	✓	Masks		Medical waste	R
Single room		Caps		Laundry	R
Private room + b/room	✓	Eye protection			
Separate equipment		Cotton gowns			
Limit visitors	✓	Plastic aprons	✓		

Legal notification		Readily communicable in the healthcare setting	
On suspicion of infection		Yes	✓
On lab confirmation		No	

R = Routine   S = Special

Comments: Impeccable hand and personal hygiene measures are required at all times. All age groups are susceptible to viral gastro-enteritis. Reinfection is possible, especially where personal hygiene and sanitation are poor. Rehydration of children and babies is essential as the accompanying dehydration may be fatal. (Refer to chapter 3, Enteric conditions (diarrhoea) on page 128.)

(Home-made rehydration fluid: 5 ml table salt, 5 ml bicarbonate of soda, and 20 ml sugar, dissolved in 1 litre of boiled, cooled water may be used as an oral rehydration solution.)

ICD-10-A07.1   GIARDIASIS *(Lambliasis, giardia enteritis)*

Signs and symptoms:	Chronic diarrhoea, steatorrhoea, bloating, abdominal cramps, fatigue, loss of weight and frequent pale loose, greasy or malodorous stools. Malabsorption and avitaminosis is common in chronic cases. The infection may also be asymptomatic. Children seldom have pyrexia.
Causative organism:	A protozoa: *Giardia lamblia.*
Method of transmission:	Faecal-oral transmission by ingesting contaminated water and food.
Incubation period:	3–25 days or even longer, generally 7 days.
Infectious period:	As long as the protozoa is present in the stools. Asymptomatic carriers are common and constitute a grave risk to others. Can last months.

CONTROL/PREVENTATIVE MEASURES

Barrier measures		Protective clothing		Housekeeping	
Hand washing	✓	Gloves	✓	Cleaning	R
Hand disinfection	✓	Masks		Medical waste	R
Single room		Caps		Laundry	R
Private room + b/room	✓	Eye protection			
Separate equipment	✓	Cotton gowns			
Limit visitors	✓	Plastic aprons	✓		

Legal notification		Readily communicable in the healthcare setting	
On suspicion of infection		Yes	✓
On lab confirmation		No	

R = Routine   S = Special

Comments: Impeccable personal hygiene is essential especially in areas where children are cared for. Unsuspecting asymptomatic adult carriers commonly and readily spread the infection to close contacts, especially children in the family and workplace. The mentally handicapped and children in day-care centers are particularly susceptible. Healthcare staff, food handlers and child minders require training and supervision to remain alert and watchful for any enteric disease in themselves, their children and colleagues. All episodes of diarrhoea (also of the family) should be reported to the worker's supervisor in order to facilitate treatment where necessary.

ICD-10-A54.3 GONOCOCCAL CONJUNCTIVITIS
(Gonorrhoeal opthalmia neonatorum)

Signs and symptoms:	Acute reddening and swelling of the conjunctiva of either one or both eyes followed by a purulent discharge. Corneal ulceration/perforation and blindness is possible if specific treatment is not administered promptly.
Causative organism:	A bacterium: *Neisseria gonorrhoea*, a gonococcus.
Method of transmission:	Contact with the infected vagina during delivery.
Incubation period:	Generally 1–5 days.
Infectious period:	As long as there is a nasal and eye discharge in untreated cases. Where effective antibiotic treatment has been administered the discharge is non-infective within 24 hours.

CONTROL/PREVENTATIVE MEASURES							
Barrier measures		**Protective clothing**		**Housekeeping**		
Hand washing	✓	Gloves	✓	Cleaning		R
Hand disinfection	✓	Masks		Medical waste		R
Incubator: 24 hours	✓	Caps		Laundry		R
Private room + b/room		Eye protection				
Separate equipment	✓	Cotton gowns				
Limit visitors	✓	Plastic aprons	✓			

Legal notification		**Readily communicable in the healthcare setting**	
On suspicion of infection		Yes	✓
On lab confirmation	✓	No	

R = Routine   S = Special

Comments: Diagnosis and treatment of the infected pregnant women is the most effective way of combating the disease and its side-effects. Isolation of infected babies, eg. by placement in a closed incubator, is only indicated for the first 24 hours after the appropriate antibiotic treatment has been started. Eye swabs should be sent for microbiological microscopy and culturing to ensure that the treatment has successfully been completed, rather than assuming that it has. The mothers of infected babies and their sexual partners should always be investigated and, if necessary, treated as well.

ICD-10-A54.0-A54.2	GONOCOCCAL INFECTION – GENITOURINARY TRACT INFECTION *(Gonorrhoea)*

Signs and symptoms: Septicaemia, painless dry or discharging skin lesions, meningitis, endocarditis and arthritis may develop in untreated patients of both sexes.
Female patients: Purulent vaginal discharge. Usually mild symptoms, often unnoticed. Infiltration of the uterus follows, leading to endometritis, salpingitis or pelvic peritonitis, and/or sterility.
Male patients: Dysuria with a purulent urethral secretion follows within 2–7 days after exposure. Epididymitis sometimes develops. Sterility may follow.

Causative organism: A bacterium: *Neisseria gonorrhoea.*

Method of transmission: Direct contact with the mucosa or contagious discharges of an infected person or sexual contact.

Incubation period: 2–7 days on average. Sometimes longer.

Infectious period: The secretions or lesions are non-infective within hours of effective antibiotic treatment being administered. In untreated cases the infection can linger for many months, especially in females. Both sexes may become chronic carriers of the disease.

CONTROL/PREVENTATIVE MEASURES					
Barrier measures		**Protective clothing**		**Housekeeping**	
Hand washing	✓	Gloves	✓	Cleaning	R
Hand disinfection	✓	Masks		Medical waste	R
Single room		Caps		Laundry	R
Private room + b/room		Eye protection			
Separate equipment	✓	Cotton gowns			
Limit visitors		Plastic aprons	✓		

Legal notification		Readily communicable in the healthcare setting	
On suspicion of infection		Yes	
On lab confirmation	✓	No	✓

R = Routine   S = Special

Comments: Sexual partners should always be treated too. Infected persons should have no sexual intercourse until the course of treatment has been completed. Good personal hygiene is essential. No work or school exclusion is necessary. Women using intrauterine contraceptive devices run a greater risk of salpingitis. After completion of a course of antibiotics, swabs or tissue specimens should be sent to the laboratory before assuming that the infection has cleared up. The eyes of babies born to untreated mothers may be infected during the delivery. This may lead to corneal lesions or even blindness. At birth, antibiotic drops should routinely be placed in a neonate's eyes. In rural areas the use of a 1% solution of silver nitrate in newborn babies' eyes is still the most common prophylactic treatment against gonorrhoea, though it may cause eye irritation.

ICD-10-B15   HEPATITIS A *(Infective or epidemic hepatitis, HAV)*

Signs and symptoms:	Onset is usually abrupt with fever, malaise, anorexia, nausea, abdominal discomfort, dark urine and clay coloured stools followed by jaundice within a few days. Varies from mild illness lasting 1–2 weeks, to longer and (rarely) several months. Convalescence is usually prolonged. Severity of disease increases with age but complete recovery is the rule. Many infections are asymptomatic or mild, without jaundice.
Causative organism:	A virus: hepatitis A virus (in faeces).
Method of transmission:	Person-to-person. Faecal-oral route after intake of contaminated food, salads and sandwiches, milk or water.
Incubation period:	15–50 days, averaging 28–30 days, depending on the infecting dose of virus.
Infectious period:	During latter half of incubation period until 1 week after jaundice has appeared. Diarrhoea may contain the virus for longer.

CONTROL/PREVENTATIVE MEASURES					
Barrier measures		**Protective clothing**		**Housekeeping**	
Hand washing	✓	Gloves	✓	Cleaning	R
Hand disinfection	✓	Masks		Medical waste	R
Single room		Caps		Laundry	R
Private room + b/room		Eye protection			
Separate equipment	✓	Cotton gowns			
Limit visitors		Plastic aprons	✓		

Legal notification		**Readily communicable in the healthcare setting**	
On suspicion of infection		Yes	
On lab confirmation	✓	No	✓

R = Routine   S = Special

Comments: If the patient is independent and can maintain a good standard of personal hygiene while using communal bathroom facilities, isolation in a private room with a bathroom is unnecessary. Immune globulin is available for administering in exceptional cases, e.g. where a number of staff have been exposed to possible infection at the same time. Acquired homologous immunity lasts for life. Children, mentally impaired persons in institutions, and people living in hostels with a communal kitchen are most susceptible because of close proximity and possible poor hygiene. Overcrowding and poor sanitation contribute to the spread of HAV. Observe contacts for symptoms and treat accordingly. Work/school exclusion is applicable until 7 days after the appearance of jaundice.

ICD-10-B16 HEPATITIS B *(Serum hepatitis, Australian antigen, HBV)*

Signs and symptoms:	Gradual onset with nausea, vomiting, abdominal discomfort, anorexia, normal or slightly elevated temperature, and jaundice. Cases may vary from mild to severe attacks resulting in hepatic necrosis. Asymptomatic or very mild attacks have been noted. HBV carriers do not always have a definite history of clinical infection. Fever may be absent or mild.
Causative organism:	A virus: hepatitis B virus (transmitted by blood and sexual secretions).
Method of transmission:	Blood and all blood products (including plasma, thrombin and packed cells); sexual secretions, especially semen, urine and saliva are contagious. Sexual contact as well as percutaneous inoculation with contaminated sharp devices such as needles and blood/blood products are the most common routes of transmission of HBV. Intrauterine transmission to an unborn foetus is probable if the mother carries the virus. Communally used razors and toothbrushes are occasional vehicles of transmission.
Incubation period:	42–180 days, on average 60–90 days.
Infectious period:	Several weeks before the first symptoms appear, during the acute stage of infection and for an unspecified time afterwards. A chronic carrier stage may develop, during which HBV may be transmissible for years.

CONTROL/PREVENTATIVE MEASURES

Barrier measures		Protective clothing		Housekeeping	
Hand washing	✓	Gloves	✓	Cleaning	R
Hand disinfection	✓	Masks		Medical waste	R
Single room		Caps		Laundry	R
Private room + b/room		Eye protection			
Separate equipment	✓	Cotton gowns			
Limit visitors		Plastic aprons	✓		

Legal notification		Readily communicable in the healthcare setting	
On suspicion of infection		Yes	
On lab confirmation	✓	No	✓

R = Routine   S = Special

Comments: All persons who are HBsAg-positive are potentially infectious. If the patient is independent and can maintain a good standard of personal hygiene while using communal bathroom facilities, isolation in a private room with a bathroom is unnecessary. Effective immunisation is available. The course must be completed following a set schedule. Immunisation of the sex partners of patients with HBV infection is strongly recommended. HBV may cause up to 80% of all hepatic carcinomas diagnosed on oncology wards. Perinatal HBV infection (before, during or just after birth) shows a high risk for the development of the chronic carrier stage. HBV infection may lead to chronic hepatitis, liver cirrhosis or primary liver carcinoma in susceptible adults. Persons who routinely come into contact with blood and human secretions should always take additional precautions. High-risk groups such as intravenous drug users, people with numerous sexual partners, as well as healthcare staff with direct exposure to the illness during patient and child care, show a higher incidence of infection than the rest of the population. HBV may be transmitted through blood transfusion, although the modern screening tests used in South Africa to exclude donated HBV positive blood are very effective. Contaminated syringes and needles, intravenous devices as well as other items that come into contact with human tissue/blood, such as tattooing equipment and ink, are known to be implicated in the spread of infection through prick accidents and careless handling. As little as 0,0004 millilitres of blood is needed to transmit HBV (while HIV needs +/-0,1 millilitres of blood). School/work exclusion for adults and teenagers is unnecessary as long as good personal hygiene is ensured (including thorough hand-washing and careful use of public toilet facilities). Children and toddlers should preferably stay at home until the most overt symptoms have disappeared.

Interpretation of positive laboratory results:

+ HBsAg = Acute infection
+ HBeAg = Chronic carrier, highly infectious
+ Anti-HBs = Immunity
+ Anti-HBc = Exposed to HBV, but insufficient antigen has yet developed
+ Anti-HBe = Carrier, but a lower level of contagiousness.

ICD-10-B17 to B19	HEPATITIS C *(Non-A, non-B hepatitis, transfusion-associated hepatitis, HCV, undifferentiated hepatitis)*

Signs and symptoms:	Insidious onset, anorexia, abdominal discomfort, nausea, vomiting, sometimes associated with jaundice. Attacks are usually mild to moderate, readily developing a chronic carrier stage (symptomatic or asymptomatic). Chronic liver disease with fluctuating or persistently elevated liver enzymes occurs in more than 60% of adult casews. There appears to be an association between HCV infection and hepato-cellular carcinoma, chronic active hepatitis and cirrhosis. Chronic infection is often asymptomatic.
Causative organism:	A virus: hepatitis C virus.
Method of transmission:	Parenteral after blood transfusion. Some patients show antibodies without ever having received blood. Used syringes and needles may also carry the virus after coming into contact with contaminated blood or plasma products. The infection may occasionally be sexually transmitted.
Incubation period:	2 weeks–6 months, averaging 6–9 weeks.
Infectious period:	A week (or more) before symptoms appear, during the acute phase of illness and lasting for an unspecified time in the chronic carrier stage. At present, research has not precisely shown how contagious HCV really is.

CONTROL/PREVENTATIVE MEASURES

Barrier measures		Protective clothing		Housekeeping	
Hand washing	✓	Gloves	✓	Cleaning	R
Hand disinfection	✓	Masks		Medical waste	R
Single room		Caps		Laundry	R
Private room + b/room		Eye protection			
Separate equipment	✓	Cotton gowns			
Limit visitors		Plastic aprons	✓		

Legal notification		Readily communicable in the healthcare setting	
On suspicion of infection		Yes	
On lab confirmation	✓	No	✓

R = Routine   S = Special

Comments: If the patient is independent and can maintain a good standard of personal hygiene while using communal bathroom facilities, isolation in a private room with a bathroom is unnecessary. Protective control/preventative measures are similar to those against HBV.

ICD-10-B00   HERPES SIMPLEX *(HSV, cold sores, blisters, human herpes virus 1 and 2)*

Signs and symptoms:	90% of primary infections with HSV type 1 are asymptomatic and occur in childhood. In the remaining 10% of primary cases, symptoms vary between a week-long fever with malaise and recurring cold sores (blisters), and encephalitis, which may lead to coma and death. Painful infection of the mucosa of the mouth and throat is common. The blisters consist of superficial clear vesicles on an erythematous base, usually on the face and lips, which crust and heal within days. Keratoconjunctivitis often occurs.
	HSV type 2 usually causes genital herpes in adults. Primary infection may be followed by repeated episodes, which may be asymptomatic. Lesions occur on the internal or external genitals.
Causative organism:	A virus: herpes simplex virus type 1 and 2.
Method of transmission:	Contact with the saliva of carriers of HSV type 1.
	Sexual contact with carriers of HSV type 2.
	The hands and fingers of healthcare staff are prone to herpetic whitlow due to contact with HSV. Transmission to the neonate during birth via the infected birth canal is possible.
Incubation period:	2–12 days.
Infectious period:	Secretion of the virus may be found for a period of up to 7 weeks after recovery from primary stomatitis lesions. Patients with genital lesions are contagious for 7–12 days after commencement of appropriate treatment. Recurring attacks usually last 4–7 days. Reactivation of the infection occurs in approximately 50% of cases and is then usually lifelong. Asymptomatic carriers readily spread the infection.

CONTROL/PREVENTATIVE MEASURES					
Barrier measures		**Protective clothing**		**Housekeeping**	
Hand washing	✓	Gloves	✓	Cleaning	R
Hand disinfection	✓	Masks		Medical waste	R
Single room	*	Caps		Laundry	R
Private room + b/room		Eye protection			
Separate equipment	✓	Cotton gowns			
Limit visitors	*	Plastic aprons	✓		

Legal notification		**Readily communicable in the healthcare setting**	
On suspicion of infection		Yes	
On lab confirmation		No	✓

*For a child   R = Routine   S = Special

Comments: Herpes blisters are reactivated by fever, disease or stress as well as immunosuppression even in the presence of circulating antibodies. Immune compromised persons are especially prone to attack. Herpes may affect other parts of the body, e.g. the gastrointestinal tract or brain (meningo-encephalitis). Normal delivery of a baby by an infected mother with active lesions carries a high risk of contamination of the newborn. A Caesarean section is usually indicated in this instance. In adult women genital herpes may be a risk factor in the development of cervical cancer. Infected patients as well as their sex partners should be taught the facts about HSV type 2 as well as the appropriate prevention/control measures. The use of good-quality latex condoms is essential as there is no definite cure, vaccine or prophylaxis available against HSV at present. Treatments that are presently available are not always successful in inhibiting the virus. No adult with HSV infection (acute or chronic) should be allowed to work with food commercially or care for children or immunosuppressed patients. School/work exclusion should be implemented during severe attacks and last until the lesions have formed a dry scab. Susceptible staff should wear gloves during contact with eczematous patients. Pregnant women should avoid contact with infected persons where possible.

ICD-10-B02   HERPES ZOSTER *(Shingles)*

Signs and symptoms:	The local acute manifestation or reactivation of latent varicella infection in the dorsal root ganglia. Vesicles form irregular patterns on the skin following the distribution of a communal sensory unilateral nerve cluster. Spinal ganglia become inflamed. Severe pain occurs in the afflicted area. The vesicles are deeper-seated and more unilaterally aggregated than those found in chickenpox. Severe pain and paresthesia are common (neuralgia).
Causative organism:	A virus: varicella zoster virus (the same type of virus that causes chickenpox, human herpes virus 3).
Method of transmission:	Contact with the vesicle fluid, respiratory secretion or contaminated fomites of infected persons.
Incubation period:	13–17 days.
Infectious period:	7 days after the appearance of the vesicles or as long as fluid is present in the vesicles. Elderly people as well as immunosuppressed persons are especially susceptible to attacks.

CONTROL/PREVENTATIVE MEASURES

Barrier measures		Protective clothing		Housekeeping	
Hand washing	✓	Gloves	✓	Cleaning	R
Hand disinfection	✓	Masks		Medical waste	R
Single room	*	Caps		Laundry	R
Private room + b/room		Eye protection			
Separate equipment	✓	Cotton gowns			
Limit visitors	*	Plastic aprons	✓		

Legal notification		Readily communicable in the healthcare setting	
On suspicion of infection		Yes	
On lab confirmation	✓	No	✓

For a child   *R = Routine   S = Special*

Comments: Staff who are not immune to chickenpox must use all the preventative measures (noted above) when working with a patient who has herpes zoster. Immune staff need only maintain a high level of hand hygiene while avoiding susceptible patients and staff members. If a person is prone to herpes zoster attacks, his/her immune status should be assessed. Persons with underlying malignancy or immune suppression (such as HIV-infection) are especially susceptible to herpes zoster. Susceptible immunosuppressed persons are considered to be contagious for 10–21 days **after** exposure. School/work exclusion lasts until all lesions have cleared up. Stress may trigger repeated attacks of herpes zoster. Scabs from varicella lesions are not infective as zoster has a lower rate of transmission than chickenpox.

ICD-10-J10/J11   INFLUENZA

Signs and symptoms:	An acute respiratory disease that presents with pyrexia, rigor, headache, myalgia, prostration, coryza and a sore throat. A severe and protracted cough follows. Nausea, vomiting and diarrhoea sometimes occur as well, especially in children. Epidemics may quickly develop, especially amongst debilitated and chronically ill patients. In healthy people the disease is usually self-limiting and recovery within 2–7 days is common, though the cough may linger for days to weeks longer.
Causative organism:	Viruses, usually influenza virus type A, B and C. Bacteria: e.g. *Haemophilus influenzae* (different subtypes).
Method of transmission:	Airborne spread in small crowded areas, as well as contact with discharged droplets of dried (evaporated) mucus.
Incubation period:	Short, generally 1–3 days.
Infectious period:	Usually 3–5 days after presentation of the initial symptoms in adults and as long as 7 days in children. The virus stays viable for hours in dried drops of mucus and may be transferred by contaminated hands from the environment to the susceptible new host.

CONTROL/PREVENTATIVE MEASURES

Barrier measures		Protective clothing		Housekeeping	
Hand washing	✓	Gloves	✓	Cleaning	R
Hand disinfection	✓	Masks		Medical waste	R
Single room		Caps		Laundry	R
Private room + b/room		Eye protection			
Separate equipment	✓	Cotton gowns			
Limit visitors		Plastic aprons	✓		

Legal notification		Readily communicable in the healthcare setting	
On suspicion of infection		Yes	✓
On lab confirmation. Only for *Haemophilus influenzae* Group B			✓

R = Routine   S = Special

Comments: Antimicrobial treatment (antibiotics) is only effective against the development of secondary bacterial infections. Vaccines against specific types of influenza are available and generally provide 70–80% protection. This may be of service in protecting elderly patients, those with chronic respiratory disorders and the healthcare staff exposed to these patients. The strains of influenza viruses differ each season and annually, which may lead to inappropriate immunisation if the strains included in the vaccine mixture have been chosen incorrectly.

Haemophilus influenzae group B may cause severe, destructive infection of the larynx, trachea and bronchi in children and debilitated older people. Sub-acute endocarditis and purulent meningitis may be caused by *H. influenzae*. Immunisation is available for paediatric patients. Infection with this specific bacterium is **notifiable by law**. Immunisation is available for paediatric patients.

ICD-10-A48.1   LEGIONELLOSIS *(Legionnaires' disease)*

Signs and symptoms:	An acute infectious disease with anorexia, pneumonia, headache, malaise, muscle and abdominal pains, fever, chills, dry cough, diarrhoea. An overall fatality rate of +/-15–39% amongst hospitalised patients is common.
Causative organism:	A bacterium: *Legionellae pneumophila.*
Method of transmission:	Airborne: spread by droplets especially from contaminated humidification equipment such as air conditioners, humidifiers and water systems.
Incubation period:	2–10 days, usually averaging 5 days.
Infectious period:	Person-to-person transfer has not been documented. Immune-compromised patients and the elderly in healthcare institutions are often affected. The bacteria can survive for lengthy periods in contaminated tap or distilled water.

CONTROL/PREVENTATIVE MEASURES

Barrier measures		Protective clothing		Housekeeping	
Hand washing	✓	Gloves	✓	Cleaning	S
Hand disinfection	✓	Masks		Medical waste	R
Single room	✓	Caps		Laundry	R
Private room + b/room		Eye protection			
Separate equipment	✓	Cotton gowns			
Limit visitors		Plastic aprons	✓		

Legal notification		Readily communicable in the healthcare setting	
On suspicion of infection		Yes	
On lab confirmation	✓	No	✓

R = Routine   S = Special

Comments: Water cooling systems and air conditioning need special cleaning, disinfection and drying after drainage of all water and fluid contents. Tracing contacts as well as sub-clinical infected persons in the community is important. Thorough epidemiological studies are indicated after even one case of the infection has been reported.

ICD-10-A30   LEPROSY *(Leprosis, Hansen's disease, lepra)*

Signs and symptoms: A chronic communicable disease characterised by lesions of the skin, upper respiratory and ocular mucous membranes, peripheral nerves and the testes. Early symptoms consist of red or brown patches on the skin, often with pale or white centers appearing later. Parts of the body supplied by these nerves may show a loss of sensation. Nodules develop, sometimes accompanied by fever. Neuritis and iritis may appear. Body hair tends to fall out.

In **lepromatous** leprosy, the nodules, papules, macules and diffuse infiltrations are bilaterally symmetrical; usually numerous and extensive. Involvement of the nasal mucosa may lead to crusting, obscured breathing and epistaxis. Ocular involvement leads to iritis and keratitis. Open sores appear on the face, earlobes and forehead. Large numbers of bacilli are found in the discharges from these lesions. In untreated cases the fingers and toes of the person disintegrate, which leads to severe disability and disfigurement. Death may follow in severe lepromatous leprosy, mostly due to secondary infections such as tuberculosis or pneumonia.

In the **tuberculoid** type of leprosy, sections of the skin show a loss of sensation as well as atrophy of the muscles. This often results in contraction of the hands into dysfunctional claws. Skin lesions are single or few, sharply demarcated anaesthetic or hypesthetic, bilaterally asymmetric.

Undifferentialised leprosy is identified as an early form of infection that later may manifest as lepromatous leprosy in a number of untreated patients, or as tuberculoid leprosy in a number of treated patients.

Causative organism: A bacterium: *Mycobacterium leprae.*

Method of transmission: Prolonged intimate household contact. Bacilli are excreted in the nasal secretions, the milk of lactating women, and from the skin lesions of untreated leprosy sufferers. Trans-placental transmission may have occurred in infected babies younger than 1 year. Tattooing has been implicated in some cases of infection.

Incubation period: 9 months to 20 years. An average of 4 years seems to be common.

Infectious period: Infectiousness is reduced after continuous treatment ranging from 3 days to 3 months, depending on the medication used. Bacilli can remain viable in dried secretions for as long as 7 days.

	CONTROL/PREVENTATIVE MEASURES				
Barrier measures		**Protective clothing**		**Housekeeping**	
Hand washing	✓	Gloves	✓	Cleaning	R
Hand disinfection	✓	Masks		Medical waste	R
Single room		Caps		Laundry	R
Private room + b/room		Eye protection			
Separate equipment	✓	Cotton gowns			
Limit visitors	✓	Plastic aprons	✓		

Legal notification		**Readily communicable in the healthcare setting**	
On suspicion of infection		Yes	
On lab confirmation	✓	No	✓

R = Routine   S = Special

Comments: Protective measures and nursing barriers are selected according to the patient's symptoms. Leprosy is endemic in southern Africa and still occurs. Overcrowding and poor socio-economic conditions promote the spread of the disease. The most likely route of entry to the host's body is through the upper respiratory tract or through broken skin, although identifying the route of either is not 100% conclusive because of the extended incubation period.

ICD-10-B50 to B52   MALARIA *(Marsh fever)*

Signs and symptoms:	Fever, rigor, sweating, disorientation, cough, convulsions, jaundice, shock, headache, liver and renal failure, acute encephalitis, blood coagulation defects, pulmonary and cerebral oedema, coma, death. Presents with malaise and a rising fever that continues for several days. Chills, profuse perspiration, severe headache and vomiting follow. After a period with no fever, the cycle repeats itself (all the symptoms reoccur daily, every alternate day or even every third day). In an untreated patient the attack may last for 1–30 days or longer. Malarial infection may persist for many years with periods as long as 2–5 years between episodes of parasitaemia.
Causative organism:	A protozoa: *Plasmodium vivax, P. falciparum, P. ovale, P. malariae.*
Method of transmission:	The bite of an infected mosquito (female *Anopheles* mosquito). Not transmittable from person-to-person, except by transfusion of contaminated blood or by sharing contaminated needles.
Incubation period:	Average 7–60 days. In some patients development may be delayed for 8-10 months (e.g. if insufficient prophylaxis has been used).
Infectious period:	As long as the infective gametocytes are present in the patient's blood. Stored (transfusion) blood may remain infective for as long as 16 days.

CONTROL/PREVENTATIVE MEASURES					
Barrier measures		**Protective clothing**		**Housekeeping**	
Hand washing	✓	Gloves	✓	Cleaning	R
Hand disinfection	✓	Masks		Medical waste	R
Single room		Caps		Laundry	R
Private room + b/room		Eye protection			
Separate equipment		Cotton gowns			
Limit visitors		Plastic aprons			

Legal notification		**Readily communicable in the healthcare setting**	
On suspicion of infection		Yes	
On lab confirmation	✓	No	✓

R = Routine   S = Special

Comments: Prophylactic treatment should commence +/-7–30 days before visiting an endemic area, depending on the specific medication, and should be taken as prescribed during the visit and kept up for at least 4 weeks after return. Permanent liver, renal and central nervous system complications are occurring more regularly and require intensive medical and nursing care, even in patients who have used prophylactic medication as specified. Mechanical ventilation and monitoring of body functions to support life are sometimes indicated. Multi-drug-resistant malaria is being encountered more frequently in southern Africa due to the increase in HIV infection, the negligence of patients in taking prophylactic medication correctly, and the failure in some countries to implement and maintain a regular combat programme against mosquitoes.

ICD-10-B05   MEASLES *(Rubeola, morbilli)*

Signs and symptoms: An extremely contagious disease. An acute onset with prodromal fever, conjunctivitis, coryza, cough, Koplik's spots on the mucosa of the mouth and throat. From day 3–7 a characteristic red macular blotchy rash appears on the face, spreading to the rest of the body, lasting an additional 4–7 days. The erythema then turns brown and starts to peel. The affliction is more severe in babies and adults than older children. Their infection usually varies from mild to moderate. Complications include ear infections, pneumonia, diarrhoea and encephalitis. Blindness, infertility, dehydration, and blood clotting abnormalities may be seen in neglected cases. The disease may be fatal in malnourished or immunosuppressed children, or children with vitamin A deficiency.

Causative organism: A virus: the measles virus, a morbilli-virus.

Method of transmission: Droplet spread (airborne) and direct contact with the nasal- and throat secretions of infected persons, indirect contact with contaminated fomites.

Incubation period: +/-10 days, averaging 7–18 days from exposure until the fever develops (prodromal period), usually 14 days until the rash appears.

Infectious period: From slightly before the start of the prodromal period to 4 days after the appearance of the rash. Active infection leads to lifelong active immunity.

CONTROL/PREVENTATIVE MEASURES					
Barrier measures		**Protective clothing**		**Housekeeping**	
Hand washing	✓	Gloves	✓	Cleaning	R
Hand disinfection	✓	Masks		Medical waste	R
Single room		Caps		Laundry	R
Private room + b/room		Eye protection			
Separate equipment	✓	Cotton gowns			
Limit visitors	✓	Plastic aprons	✓		

Legal notification		**Readily communicable in the healthcare setting**	
On suspicion of infection		Yes	✓
On lab confirmation	✓	No	

R = Routine   S = Special

Comments: Effective immunisation is available. Immunisation of contacts with immunoglobin is possible up to 6 days after exposure. Nurse in a darkened room as the patients are photophobic. Administration of therapeutic doses of vitamin A may relieve the severity of the symptoms. Immunisation administered after the third day following exposure may only extend the incubation period of the infection rather than prevent the disease. School/work exclusion is compulsory and extends to 7 days after the rash first appeared.

ICD-10-A39.0 MENINGITIS – MENINGOCOCCAL
(Bacterial meningococcal meningitis)

Signs and symptoms:	An acute disease with a sudden onset, fever, intense headache, a stiff neck, nausea, vomiting, shock and exhaustion. Sometimes a rash appears (petechiae, pink macules and/or, rarely, vesicles). Delirium and coma are characteristic. The infection may even present mildly or asymptomatically. In untreated cases the mortality rate is high, especially if pneumonia, septicaemia or meningococcaemia develops.
Causative organism:	A bacterium: *Neisseria meningitidis.*
Method of transmission:	Direct contact with the respiratory discharges of infected persons as well as through droplet spread. A +/-25% prevalence rate of asymptomatic carriers of neisseria amongst some groups in the general population is estimated (e.g. children). They act as a source of infection for new susceptible hosts.
Incubation period:	2–10 days, averaging 3–4 days.
Infectious period:	As long as the meningococci are viable in the nasal and throat discharges of infected persons. The period of contagion ends after 24 hours of effective antibiotic treatment.

CONTROL/PREVENTATIVE MEASURES

Barrier measures		Protective clothing		Housekeeping	
Hand washing	✓	Gloves	✓	Cleaning	S
Hand disinfection	✓	Masks for 48 hrs	✓	Medical waste	R
Single room		Caps for 48 hrs	✓	Laundry	R
Private room + b/room	✓	Eye protection			
Separate equipment	✓	Cotton gowns			
Limit visitors for 48 hrs	✓	Plastic aprons for 48 hrs	✓		

Legal notification		Readily communicable in the healthcare setting	
On suspicion of infection		Yes	✓
On lab confirmation	✓	No	

R = Routine   S = Special

Comments: The infection usually occurs in children and teenagers in autumn/winter and spring. **Face masks** are the most important means of protection for staff and are indicated when contact within one metre of the patient is to be maintained for a period of time. The use of face masks can be discontinued after completion of 24 hours of effective antibiotic treatment. Paediatric immunisation is available. If the organism seems to be resistant to the antibiotic the patient is being treated with, or if there is uncertainty about the suitability of the treatment, the isolation period should be extended accordingly. Adults are clinically less susceptible to the disease, leading to a larger incidence of carriers than patients amongst them. Overcrowding in living conditions or workplaces encourages the spread of the disease. Tracing contacts of patients with meningococcal meningitis is important. 'Contacts' include people who have come within one metre of the patient for a period of time, all household and family members, school-mates and anybody who may have shared eating utensils with the patient. These persons should be evaluated for pyrexia or coryza (flu-like symptoms). Prophylactic treatment must be administered as soon as possible within the first 72 hours after exposure. According to law, the local authority where the patient is resident and the Regional Director of the Department of Health have to be notified within 24 hours (by telephone) of the meningococcal meningitis diagnosis. Written documentation is to follow within 7 days. The patient may return to work or school when the doctor indicates that there is no more risk of spreading the infection (usually when all symptoms have cleared up completely).

ICD-10-39.2 to A39.8; G00	MENINGITIS *(Aseptic meningitis, bacterial/viral meningitis)*

Signs and symptoms:	Sudden onset of a febrile illness with central nervous system involvement. A red blotchy rash with varying sizes of petechiae and sometimes bleeding vesicles (viral infection) may appear. The active stage of the illness seldom exceeds 10 days. Acute headache, fever, neck stiffness, drowsiness, convulsions, nausea and vomiting are common. Delirium and coma may occur. Temporary muscle fatigue and encephalitis may last as long as a year. Recovery is (usually) complete except in frail/immunosuppressed or undernourished children and adults where the fatality rate is high.
Causative organism:	Various viruses or bacteria including the coxsackievirus, enterovirus and arboviruses. Bacteria: *Leptospira, pneumococci, streptococcus* and *haemophilus*.
Method of transmission:	Droplet spread or direct contact with secretions from the nose, throat and mouth of infected persons/carriers. In some patients organisms may be transferred by direct contact with wound discharges after head injuries or brain surgery.
Incubation period:	Indeterminable, depending on the causative organism. Usually 2–7 days at the least.
Infectious period:	As long as viable organisms are present in the secretions. Laboratory culture and sensitivity results are necessary for bacterial identification before commencing antibiotic treatment for bacterial meningitis.

CONTROL/PREVENTATIVE MEASURES

Barrier measures		Protective clothing		Housekeeping	
Hand washing	✓	Gloves	✓	Cleaning	S
Hand disinfection	✓	Masks for 48 hrs	✓	Medical waste	R
Single room for 48 hrs	✓	Caps	✓	Laundry	R
Private room + b/room		Eye protection			
Separate equipment	✓	Cotton gowns			
Limit visitors for 48 hrs	✓	Plastic aprons	✓		

Legal notification		Readily communicable in the healthcare setting	
On suspicion of infection		Yes	
On lab confirmation		No	✓

R = Routine   S = Special

Comments: The infection usually occurs in young people. HIV-positive persons have an especially high risk of contracting the disease in overcrowded settings. Various diseases such as infective mononucleosis, tuberculosis, syphilis and insufficiently/unsuitably treated septic meningitis may resemble aseptic meningitis. The aftermath of viral diseases such as measles, chickenpox,

73

hepatitis and mumps as well as inoculation against rabies or smallpox may give rise to similar signs and symptoms as aseptic meningitis. The identification of the causative organism determines which preventative/control measures are to be initiated. Until this is done, **all** cases of suspected meningitis must be nursed using face masks as if meningococcal in origin.

ICD-10-B27   MONONUCLEOSIS *(Glandular fever)*

Signs and symptoms:	An acute disease characterised by fever, sore throat, and an inflammatory swelling of the lymph nodes, especially of the cervical area. The blood analysis shows an abnormal increase of the leucocytes and lymphocytes.
Causative organism:	A virus: Epstein-Barr virus (EBV, human herpes virus 4).
Method of transmission:	Intimate contact with the saliva of a patient, contaminated hands/fomites as well as blood transfusion.
Incubation period:	4–6 weeks.
Infectious period:	A prolonged period: pharyngeal excretion may persist for a year after the acute infection has cleared up. 15–20% or more of healthy adults are long-term oropharyngeal carriers.

CONTROL/PREVENTATIVE MEASURES					
Barrier measures		**Protective clothing**		**Housekeeping**	
Hand washing	✓	Gloves	✓	Cleaning	R
Hand disinfection	✓	Masks		Medical waste	R
Single room		Caps		Laundry	R
Private room + b/room		Eye protection			
Separate equipment	✓	Cotton gowns			
Limit visitors		Plastic aprons	✓		

Legal notification		**Readily communicable in the healthcare setting**	
On suspicion of infection		Yes	
On lab confirmation		No	✓

R = Routine   S = Special

Comments: It is advisable to wash hands after contact with oral secretions, and avoid drinking from a common or communal container in order to limit contact with saliva.

ICD-10-A43   NOCARDIOSIS

Signs and symptoms:	A chronic disease, commonly originating in the lungs, usually spread through the bloodstream, producing abscesses in the brain, subcutaneous tissue and other organs. Immune-compromised patients are most susceptible to the infection, especially renal dialysis patients and persons on steroid or cytotoxic therapy. The infection carries a high mortality rate, except in cases of subcutaneous involvement.
Causative organism:	A bacterium: *Nocardia asteroides* or *N. brasiliensis*; aerobic actinomycetes.
Method of transmission:	Direct contact with abscesses or oral secretions of infected persons; inhalation of contaminated dust.
Incubation period:	Uncertain. Probably days or weeks, depending on the infecting dosage of organisms and the immune status of the patient.
Infectious period:	A contaminated environment may infect a susceptible patient. It is unknown how long the bacteria remain viable in the environment as this depends on other factors (such as hygiene) as well. Not directly transmitted from person-to-person.

CONTROL/PREVENTATIVE MEASURES

Barrier measures		Protective clothing		Housekeeping	
Hand washing	✓	Gloves	✓	Cleaning	S
Hand disinfection	✓	Masks	✓	Medical waste	R
Single room	✓	Caps		Laundry	R
Private room + b/room		Eye protection			
Separate equipment	✓	Cotton gowns			
Limit visitors		Plastic aprons	✓		

Legal notification		Readily communicable in the healthcare setting	
On suspicion of infection		Yes	
On lab confirmation		No	✓

R = Routine   S = Special

Comments: Patients on mechanical ventilators are at risk of acquiring this infection. Healthcare staff and visitors can readily spread the infection by temporarily carrying the organism in the nasopharynx. A contaminated environment may remain a constant source of infection for susceptible future patients.

ICD-10-A01.1 to A01.4   **PARATYPHOID FEVER** *(Enteric fever)*

Signs and symptoms:	A systemic disease presenting with fever, headache, malaise, anorexia, bradycardia, an enlarged spleen, a dry cough, diarrhoea in children and constipation in adults, and enlarged lymph nodes. Sometimes rose-coloured spots appear on the trunk. The infection may also be asymptomatic.
Causative organism:	A bacterium: *Salmonella paratyphi*, group A, B and C.
Method of transmission:	Food and water are contaminated by infected urine or stool, especially shellfish, raw vegetables and fruit, milk and other dairy products which are easily contaminated. Flies may spread the infection by infecting food.
Incubation period:	1–10 days, depending on the size of the infecting dose of bacteria.
Infectious period:	From the time of infection, as long as the bacilli are present in the excreta, until the condition has cleared completely (usually 1–2 weeks). 2–5% of patients become permanent carriers (in the blood, gut, urinary tract and gall-bladder).

CONTROL/PREVENTATIVE MEASURES					
Barrier measures		**Protective clothing**		**Housekeeping**	
Hand washing	✓	Gloves	✓	Cleaning	R
Hand disinfection	✓	Masks		Medical waste	R
Single room		Caps		Laundry	R
Private room + b/room		Eye protection			
Separate equipment	✓	Cotton gowns			
Limit visitors		Plastic aprons	✓		

Legal notification		**Readily communicable in the healthcare setting**	
On suspicion of infection		Yes	
On lab confirmation		No	✓

R = Routine   S = Special

Comments: If the patient is independent and can maintain a good standard of personal hygiene while using communal bathroom facilities, isolation in a private room with a bathroom is unnecessary. Family members often become temporary carriers. More chronic carriers develop among older infected persons. Good personal habits and hand hygiene are important in combating the spread of the disease. Contacts need to be evaluated microbiologically to ensure that they are not infected. School/work exclusion lasts until all symptoms have cleared up. Three negative stool and urine cultures are indicative of recovery. Specimens are collected 24 hours apart and 48 hours after the last antibiotic was administered. No completely effective immunisation against paratyphoid is available.

ICD-10-B26   PAROTITIS *(Mumps, infectious parotitis)*

Signs and symptoms:	An acute infectious disease characterised by fever, headache, tenderness and swelling of one or more salivary glands, usually the parotid and sometimes the sublingual or submaxillary glands. Unilateral orchitis occurs in 20–30% of post-pubescent males and oophoritis in +/-5% of females past puberty. Complications of mumps include meningitis and possible permanent unilateral nerve deafness.
Causative organism:	A virus: mumps virus *(paramyxovirus)*.
Method of transmission:	Droplet spread as well as direct contact with the saliva of an infected person. Inapparent infection is not uncommon and can be transmitted.
Incubation period:	12–25 days, average 18 days. Most infectious 48 hours before onset of the illness. General infectiousness commences 6–7 days before overt parotitis and extends another 9 days afterwards. Urine may stay positive for as long as 14 days after the onset of the illness. Convalescence may require as long as 25 days.

CONTROL/PREVENTATIVE MEASURES

Barrier measures		Protective clothing		Housekeeping	
Hand washing	✓	Gloves	✓	Cleaning	S
Hand disinfection	✓	Masks	✓	Medical waste	R
Single room	✓	Caps		Laundry	R
Private room + b/room		Eye protection			
Separate equipment	✓	Cotton gowns			
Limit visitors	✓	Plastic aprons	✓		

Legal notification		Readily communicable in the healthcare setting	
On suspicion of infection		Yes	✓
On lab confirmation		No	

R = Routine   S = Special

Comments: The incidence of spontaneous abortion during the first trimester of pregnancy increases after infection with mumps. Immunisation is available for use after 15 months of age in unexposed persons. Hyper-immune globuline is available to treat exposed persons. Infectiousness decreases after the appearance of the symptoms. Work/school exclusion extends until 9 days after the appearance of the swollen glands. Observe the contacts of the infected person for symptoms and treat symptomatically. Children and teenagers are particularly susceptible to infection.

ICD-10-B85   PEDICULOSIS *(Louse infestation)*

Signs and symptoms:	Infestation of the head, hairy parts of the body or sometimes the clothing, especially the seams, with adult lice, larvae or nits (eggs). Severe itching, excoriation of the scalp or scratches may lead to secondary infection. Body lice may cause typhus, trench fever and relapsing fever.
Causative organism:	*Pediculus humanus capitis* (the head louse), *P. humanis corporis* (the body louse) and *Phthirus pubis* (the pubic louse).
Method of transmission:	Direct contact with an infested person or indirectly by contact with personal belongings such as contaminated clothing; by sharing combs and caps. Pubic lice are usually transmitted through sexual contact.
Incubation period:	Under optimum conditions the eggs hatch within a week and sexual maturity is reached in +/-8–10 days.
Infectious period:	As long as lice or eggs remain viable on the infested person and/or clothing. Head and body lice can survive for a week without a food source.

CONTROL/PREVENTATIVE MEASURES							
Barrier measures		**Protective clothing**		**Housekeeping**		
Hand washing	✓	Gloves	✓	Cleaning		R
Hand disinfection	✓	Masks		Medical waste		R
Single room		Caps		Laundry		R
Private room + b/room		Eye protection				
Separate equipment	✓	Cotton gowns				
Limit visitors		Plastic aprons	✓			

Legal notification		**Readily communicable in the healthcare setting**	
On suspicion of infection		Yes	
On lab confirmation		No	✓

R = Routine   S = Special

Comments: Avoid physical contact with the patient (isolate) for at least 24 hours after an effective insecticidal shampoo has been used on the skin and all the clothes have been changed. The manufacturer's instructions must be followed precisely. Repeat after 24 hours if necessary. The clothes, bed linen and personal belongings of a person infested with body lice must be washed with warm water and soap or dry-cleaned. All intimate contacts (family members, other children in crèches/nursery schools) must be examined and treated if necessary. School/work exclusion is indicated until the infested person is free of nits. Persons infested with head and body lice may need a repeat of the treatment after 7–10 days to ensure that no nits have survived. Certain products must be used with extreme care by pregnant women and on babies and toddlers – consult the manufacturer's instructions.

ICD-10-A37.9   PERTUSSIS *(Whooping cough)*

Signs and symptoms:	An acute respiratory infection involving the tracheo-bronchial tree. The catarrhal stage has an insidious onset with mild fever, malaise and an irritating cough, which gradually becomes paroxysmal within 1–2 weeks. During this stage the cough increases in intensity, ending in the characteristic inspiratory 'whoop'. This stage may last 2–3 months, especially if pneumonia develops. The mortality rate is high amongst unimmunised babies and children. The mucous secretion is tenacious and usually clear. Vomiting generally follows coughing.
Causative organism:	A bacterium: *Borditella pertussis.*
Method of transmission:	Direct contact with secretions as well as droplet spread. Spreads readily in the intimate confines of a household.
Incubation period:	6–20 days, average14 days.
Infectious period:	Highly contagious during the early catarrhal stage, up to 3 weeks after onset of the paroxysmal stage. If the person receives antimicrobial therapy, the communicable period is reduced to 5–7 days.

CONTROL/PREVENTATIVE MEASURES

Barrier measures		Protective clothing		Housekeeping	
Hand washing	✓	Gloves	✓	Cleaning	R
Hand disinfection	✓	Masks	✓	Medical waste	R
Single room		Caps	✓	Laundry	R
Private room + b/room	✓	Eye protection			
Separate equipment	✓	Cotton gowns			
Limit visitors	✓	Plastic aprons	✓		

Legal notification		Readily communicable in the healthcare setting	
On suspicion of infection		Yes	
On lab confirmation	✓	No	✓

R = Routine   S = Special

Comments: Active immunisation is recommended for children. Unimmunised family contacts younger than 7 years may return to school or crèches/pre-school after 2 weeks from the time of exposure. Isolation need only last 5 days if the patient and contacts are given appropriate antibiotics. Antibiotics only shorten the period of contagion, and often have little effect on the symptoms unless administered during the incubation period or early stage of infection.

ICD-10-A20   PLAGUE *(Pestilence/pestis)*

Signs and symptoms:	An acute febrile infection with moderate fatality rate. Presents with acute fever, chills, nausea, vomiting, sore throat, toxaemia, petechiae, haemorrhage in the subcutaneous tissues and organs, constipation followed by diarrhoea, swollen lymphnodes and septicaemia when the infection spreads to various organs and systems. Various forms of plague are found: **Pestis minor** is a mild localised infection of short duration. **Pneumonic plague** (the most contagious form) has the most side-effects and is readily spread by airborne droplets. Untreated **septicaemic** and pneumonic plague is mostly fatal. **Bubonic** plague has a fatality rate of +/-50% in untreated cases. Septicaemia with infected draining lymph nodes (buboes) is common in bubonic plague (the 'Black Death'), followed by a necrotic rash appearing from the third day. The development of secondary 'super infections' is common.
Causative organism:	A bacterium – *Yersinia pestis.*
Method of transmission:	The bite of a flea from an infected rat or mouse or contact with the secretions of draining buboes/contaminated clothing or bed linen. Pneumonic plague spreads form person-to-person (airborne). Pets such as rabbits and cats can carry the fleas.
Incubation period:	1–8 days.
Infectious period:	Contagious as long as viable bacteria are present in secretions. Under suitable conditions, infected fleas may live from weeks to months. Overcrowding encourages the spread of pneumonic plague.

CONTROL/PREVENTATIVE MEASURES

Barrier measures		Protective clothing		Housekeeping	
Hand washing	✓	Gloves	✓	Cleaning	R
Hand disinfection	✓	Masks	✓	Medical waste	R
Single room	✓	Caps		Laundry	S
Private room + b/room		Eye protection			
Separate equipment	✓	Cotton gowns			
Limit visitors	✓	Plastic aprons	✓		

Legal notification		Readily communicable in the healthcare setting	
On suspicion of infection		Yes	
On lab confirmation	✓	No	✓

R = Routine   S = Special

Comments: A vaccine is available for use in endemic areas or for the treatment of close contacts. Rid the environment of fleas by regular and correct use of insecticides. With appropriate antibiotic treatment the patient usually improves within 24–48 hours. Bubonic plague is reasonably treatable with modern medicine. Pneumonic and septicaemic plague respond positively if the condition is diagnosed early. Home quarantine (as well as school and work exclusion) of 7 days is appropriate for close contacts of the patient. They should all be given prophylactic treatment. Tracing contacts in the community is very important. Fever may recur due to the suppuration of buboes or the development of secondary infections. Overcrowding, poor sanitation and insufficient control of rodents may cause episodes of plague that are the forerunners of epidemics.

ICD-10-A80   POLIOMYELITIS *(Infantile paralysis)*

Signs and symptoms:	An acute viral disease that varies from mild asymptomatic infection to aseptic meningitis, severe paralytic disease and possibly death. Symptoms include fever, headache, nausea, vomiting, stiffness of the neck and back, with or without flaccid paralysis, most commonly of the lower extremities. Paralysis of the muscles controlling respiration and swallowing may be life-threatening. The site of the paralysis depends on the location of the nerve cell destruction in the spinal cord or brain stem, but is always asymmetrical and reached in 3–4 days.
Causative organism:	A virus: The polio virus type 1, 2 and 3.
Method of transmission:	Droplet spread is common. Direct contact with throat secretions, and faecal-oral spread if persons live in overcrowded conditions.
Incubation period:	3–35 days, average 7–14 days in paralytic cases.
Infectious period:	The virus is present in the throat for 7 days before symptoms appear and remains in the stools for 3–6 weeks. Cases are most infectious during the first few days after onset of the symptoms.

CONTROL/PREVENTATIVE MEASURES

Barrier measures		Protective clothing		Housekeeping	
Hand washing	✓	Gloves	✓	Cleaning	S
Hand disinfection	✓	Masks		Medical waste	R
Single room		Caps		Laundry	S
Private room + b/room	✓	Eye protection			
Separate equipment	✓	Cotton gowns			
Limit visitors	✓	Plastic aprons	✓		

Legal notification		Readily communicable in the healthcare setting	
On suspicion of infection		Yes	
On lab confirmation	✓	No	✓

R = Routine   S = Special

Comments: Confirmation of the diagnosis by blood and stool analysis is extremely important, as polio is considered to be practically eradicated in South Africa. Effective polio vaccines are available. Establish whether the patient's family members have been immunised. Enteric spread is possible in children. The patient is supported symptomatically as no further treatment is available. Physiotherapy to prevent drop foot due to paralysis of the limbs is indicated. Acute-stage bulbar poliomyelitis (affecting respiration and swallowing) may necessitate critical care and mechanical ventilation. Work/school exclusion lasts until the doctor gives the patient a clean bill of health. All patients 15 years and younger, diagnosed with Guillain-Barré syndrome must be assessed for polio as well. As a precaution, all cases of acute flaccid paralysis must be reported to the local Department of Health for polio assessment.

ICD-10-A82   RABIES *(Hydrophobia)*

Signs and symptoms:	An acute encephalomyelitis that is usually fatal within 2–6 days. Headache, fever, malaise, a sense of apprehension, hyper-salivation, indefinite sensory changes (especially in the site of a preceding animal bite wound). Paresis or paralysis of the muscles may develop, and delirium and convulsions follow. Attempts to swallow cause muscle spasms and the fear of drinking (hydrophobia). Death is often due to respiratory paralysis.
Causative organism:	A rhabdovirus: the rabies virus.
Method of transmission:	The bite of a rabid animal. The virus is present in the saliva of infected animals – usually dogs, jackals, rats or meerkats (mongooses). Theoretically person-to-person transmission is possible, as the virus is present in an infected person's saliva. The virus slowly migrates along the nerve tissue to the brain.
Incubation period:	Usually 3–8 weeks. Sometimes as short as 9 days or as long as 12 months, depending on the severity and site of the wound (in relation to the richness of the nerve supply as well as the distance from the brain), the infecting dose of virus introduced, and the treatment given after exposure.
Infectious period:	3–10 days in people, dogs and cats before the onset of clinical signs and symptoms; during the acute phase of the infection until death. May vary according to circumstances.

CONTROL/PREVENTATIVE MEASURES

Barrier measures		Protective clothing		Housekeeping	
Hand washing	✓	Gloves	✓	Cleaning	S
Hand disinfection	✓	Masks	✓	Medical waste	R
Single room		Caps	✓	Laundry	S
Private room + b/room	✓	Eye protection	✓		
Separate equipment	✓	Cotton gowns			
Limit visitors	✓	Plastic aprons			

Legal notification		Readily communicable in the healthcare setting	
On suspicion of infection		Yes	
On lab confirmation	✓	No	✓

R = Routine   S = Special

Comments: Healthcare workers and family members must protect themselves from exposure when in contact with any of the patient's nasal or throat secretions. Be aware of behavioural changes in animals: for example, tame animals that suddenly appear wild/excessively restless, or wild animals that seem tame; anorexia; excessive salivation; inability to swallow or drink. All pets should be immunised against rabies.

After-exposure prophylaxis: When an animal bite or scratch has broken the skin, the wound should be vigorously washed with soap and warm water to clean it and encourage bleeding, then flushed with running water to retard blood coagulation. Suturing should be delayed unless unavoidable for cosmetic reasons or to support tissues. The patient **must** see a doctor or go to a hospital without delay, as all animal bites do need treatment, no matter how slight. Rabies immune globulin (RIG) must be administered to the patient as soon as possible after exposure in order to neutralise the virus in the tissue. This is supplemented by vaccine that is administered to a set roster per kilogram body weight, in order to encourage the development of active immunity. Administration of tetanus prophylaxis and antibiotics at the same time is recommended as well.

ICD-10-A100 to A102   RHEUMATIC FEVER *(Acute rheumatic fever)*

Signs and symptoms:	An acute inflammatory disease that presents 2–3 weeks after an episode of streptococcal infection (sore throat, upper respiratory tract or ear infection). Symptoms include fever, vague discomfort of the limbs, nosebleeds, and swollen and tender joints. The severity of the pain in the joints varies, often subsiding before moving to another location. During the acute phase, the body temperature may reach 40°C. This phase usually varies from 10–14 days. A rash may appear. Glandular nodules may be felt or seen under the skin of the elbow, knee or wrist joints. Several months after the initial infection, some patients develop spasmodic and involuntary movements known as Sydenham's chorea. Complications of rheumatic fever include developing heart valve incompetence or heart murmurs, with chronic rheumatic fever as the end result.
Causative organism:	A bacterium: *Streptococcus pyogenes* (beta-haemolytic streptococcus Group A).
Method of transmission:	Direct or intimate contact with an infective patient or carrier. Nasal carriers are often unaware of being infected. In fact, rheumatic fever is only a complication of the primary infection.
Incubation period:	1–7 days.
Infectious period:	Acute rheumatic fever is not transmittable. The primary streptococcal infection may continue for several days to weeks if left untreated. The contagiousness of untreated carriers usually spontaneously decreases within 2–3 weeks. If appropriate antibiotics are given, the contagion ends within 24–48 hours.

CONTROL/PREVENTATIVE MEASURES					
Barrier measures		**Protective clothing**		**Housekeeping**	
Hand washing	✓	Gloves	✓	Cleaning	R
Hand disinfection	✓	Masks		Medical waste	R
Single room		Caps		Laundry	R
Private room + b/room		Eye protection			
Separate equipment	✓	Cotton gowns			
Limit visitors		Plastic aprons	✓		

Legal notification		**Readily communicable in the healthcare setting**	
On suspicion of infection		Yes	
On lab confirmation	✓	No	✓

R = Routine   S = Special

Comments: Acute rheumatic fever need only be reported to the local Health Authority once. If rheumatic fever presents with complications such as heart murmur or valve incompetence, it is rather classified as rheumatic heart disease. Streptococcal sore throat can take on epidemic proportions after the intake of contaminated food such as milk, dairy products and boiled eggs. Identification of nasal carriers in general is usually a futile exercise – the biological load of the micro-organism in the nasal passages of a carrier differs on consecutive days and even at different times of the day.

ICD-10-B35   RINGWORM OF THE SKIN *(Tinea)*

Signs and symptoms:	An infectious disease of the skin, presenting as flat ring-shaped lesions that spread readily. The border is usually reddish; the surface is either vesicular or pustular, dry and scaly, or moist and encrusted. The lesions leave permanent bald patches on the scalp (tinea capitis) as the infected hair becomes brittle and falls out.
Causative organism:	A fungus: most commonly a species of *Microsporum* or *Trichophyton*.
Method of transmission:	Direct or indirect contact with lesions or hair from infected persons, animals, or contaminated fomites such as brushes, combs, chair backs, pillows or clothing.
Incubation period:	10–14 days.
Infectious period:	As long as the viable fungus is present on contaminated fomites, or in skin lesions.

CONTROL/PREVENTATIVE MEASURES

Barrier measures		Protective clothing		Housekeeping	
Hand washing	✓	Gloves	✓	Cleaning	S
Hand disinfection	✓	Masks		Medical waste	R
Single room	✓	Caps		Laundry	S
Private room + b/room		Eye protection			
Separate equipment	✓	Cotton gowns			
Limit visitors	✓	Plastic aprons	✓		

Legal notification		Readily communicable in the healthcare setting	
On suspicion of infection		Yes	
On lab confirmation		No	✓

R = Routine   S = Special

Comments: Good personal hygiene is essential to combat the infection. Pets such as cats and dogs may become inapparent carriers of the fungus. Secondary infection may follow if lesions become infected.

ICD-10- B06   RUBELLA *(German measles)*

Signs and symptoms:	A highly communicable disease with mild fever, headache, mild coryza, conjunctivitis and malaise. A diffuse reddish macular rash appears on the face and trunk. From the second day it spreads to the limbs. The lymph nodes in the neck and head start swelling a week prior to the appearance of the rash. The rash usually lasts 4 days. Congenital rubella syndrome occurs in babies whose mothers contract rubella in the first trimester of pregnancy. Intrauterine death, spontaneous abortion, and various congenital defects of the organs of the newborn are all common. Deafness and blindness, jaundice, heart defects and congenital glaucoma may occur as well.
Causative organism:	A virus: rubella virus.
Method of transmission:	Droplet spread and direct contact with the nasopharyngeal discharges of an infected person.
Incubation period:	14–23 days.
Infectious period:	From 1 week before until 5 days after onset of the rash. Infants with congenital rubella syndrome may shed the virus via their urine and nasal secretions for months after birth.

CONTROL/PREVENTATIVE MEASURES

Barrier measures		Protective clothing		Housekeeping	
Hand washing	✓	Gloves	✓	Cleaning	S
Hand disinfection	✓	Masks	✓	Medical waste	R
Single room		Caps		Laundry	R
Private room + b/room	✓	Eye protection			
Separate equipment	✓	Cotton gowns			
Limit visitors	✓	Plastic aprons	✓		

Legal notification		Readily communicable in the healthcare setting	
On suspicion of infection		Yes	✓
On lab confirmation		No	

R = Routine S = Special

Comments: Staff members that are immune to rubella may care for patients without the need for protective clothing such as face masks. As always, good hand hygiene is indicated. A vaccine is available, but is not indicated for use in pregnant women or immunosuppressed patients. In cases of natural infection during the first trimester, termination of pregnancy is usually considered. Staff members working in paediatric care units or maternity wards should be immunised against rubella. Immune globulin administered to exposed persons only suppresses the symptoms, but will not necessarily prevent the development of the disease after exposure. Work/school exclusion is indicated until 7 days after the onset of the rash.

ICD-10-A02   SALMONELLOSIS

Signs and symptoms: An acute enterocolitis with sudden onset of headache, abdominal pain, diarrhoea, nausea and sometimes vomiting. Dehydration may be severe, with anorexia and diarrhoea persisting for several days. The infection may develop into septicaemia or a focal point of sepsis. Abscesses and complications such as cholecystitis, endocarditis, pneumonia or arthritis may present. Deaths are uncommon, except in very young, debilitated or elderly patients. Asymptomatic carriers may spread the infection.

Causative organism: A bacteria: different serotypes of *Salmonella*, but mostly *Salmonella* group B.

Method of transmission: Ingestion of contaminated food, such as raw or under-cooked eggs and egg products, milk and dairy products, meat and poultry. Faecal-oral transmission from person-to-person is common if diarrhoea is present, especially in children or mentally handicapped persons.

Incubation period: 6–72 hours, average 12–36 hours.

Infectious period: Usually several days, even weeks. A temporary carrier stage may last for months. Toddlers may secrete the bacteria for up to a year. After the administration of antibiotics, the period of communicability may be extended – even with the appropriate antimicrobial treatment.

CONTROL/PREVENTATIVE MEASURES					
Barrier measures		**Protective clothing**		**Housekeeping**	
Hand washing	✓	Gloves	✓	Cleaning	S
Hand disinfection	✓	Masks		Medical waste	R
Single room		Caps		Laundry	R
Private room + b/room	✓	Eye protection			
Separate equipment	✓	Cotton gowns			
Limit visitors	✓	Plastic aprons	✓		

Legal notification		**Readily communicable in the healthcare setting**	
On suspicion of infection		Yes	✓
On lab confirmation		No	

R = Routine   S = Special

Comments: Hospitals and other healthcare facilities caring for debilitated persons run a real risk of the outbreak of salmonellosis, as the organism remains viable in the environment for lengthy periods of time. Reinfection from this source is possible, and usually starts with contaminated food and then spreads from person-to-person via the staff's hands and contaminated equipment. Non-chlorinated water sources in the community may be contaminated and can rapidly cause an epidemic. The routine use of raw eggs should be avoided and only clean, unbroken eggs bought. Work/school exclusion is indicated until all symptoms have disappeared, even though the organism may remain viable in the stools for weeks to months. Sufferers and their families must be educated in maintaining high standards of basic personal hygiene, and especially handwashing. Overcrowding and poor sanitation promote the spread of salmonellosis.

ICD-10-B86   SCABIES *(Ascariasis, sarcoptic itch)*

Signs and symptoms:	An infestation caused by a parasitic mite that penetrates the skin. The parasites are visible in children as small papules/vesicles in tiny linear burrows containing the mites and eggs. Lesions in the body folds, at the wrists and elbows and around the nails harbour the mite and its burrows. In babies, the soft skin of the neck, palms, soles of feet and head are usually infested as well. Intense itching occurs, especially at night, but the most severe complications stem from secondary infections caused by scratching and breaking the skin.
Causative organism:	A mite – *Sarcoptes scabei.*
Method of transmission:	Direct contact with the infested skin; to a lesser extent, contact with contaminated clothing and bed linen. Sexual transmission due to contact.
Incubation period:	2–6 weeks before itching commences in persons not previously infested. Persons previously infested and sensitised develop symptoms within 1–4 days after re-exposure.
Infectious period:	Until all viable mites and eggs are destroyed – usually after 1–2 treatments a week apart.

CONTROL/PREVENTATIVE MEASURES

Barrier measures		Protective clothing		Housekeeping	
Hand washing	✓	Gloves	✓	Cleaning	R
Hand disinfection	✓	Masks		Medical waste	R
Single room	✓	Caps		Laundry	S
Private room + b/room		Eye protection			
Separate equipment	✓	Cotton gowns			
Limit visitors		Plastic aprons	✓		

Legal notification		Readily communicable in the healthcare setting	
On suspicion of infection		Yes	✓
On lab confirmation		No	

R = Routine   S = Special

Comments: Contaminated persons are excluded from work/school for 24 hours after the onset of treatment. Clothing and bed linen used during the previous 48 hours, before commencing treatment, must be washed with hot water and soap and hung out in the sun. After bathing with a specially prescribed lotion, the afflicted person must change into clean clothing. Itching may persist for 1–2 weeks in spite of the treatment. In +/-5% of cases, a second course of treatment within 7–10 days may be needed. Some of the lotions are extremely toxic so over-treatment must be avoided. Intimate contacts of afflicted persons should be traced and examined. Educating the whole family about good personal hygiene is necessary to ensure that they remain free of infestation. Regular inspection of day-care centers, crèches, homeless shelters and institutions caring for the elderly and mentally handicapped should be undertaken.

ICD-10-A38   SCARLET FEVER

Signs and symptoms:	This is not a true infection: the skin rash develops due to the patient's sensitivity to the exotoxin secreted by the infecting streptococci.
	Fever, sore throat, septic tonsillitis and pharyngitis, a red rash, tender and swollen glands as well as nausea and vomiting are common. The palate, tonsils and pharynx may be red and swollen, and raised petechiae are usually seen on the flushed mucosa. The bright red exanthema – usually on the neck, chest, axilla, elbows and insides of the thighs – feels like fine sandpaper, and pales when pressure is applied. Although the rash does not appear on the face, the patient's cheeks are flushed, with circumoral pallor. The rash fades in about a week. The strawberry-red tongue is very characteristic. During recovery, the skin of the finger- and toe tips, the soles of the feet and palms of the hands peels off. Late complications of streptococcal infections include conditions such as sub-acute bacterial endocarditis and rheumatic fever.
Causative organism:	A bacterium: *Streptococcus pyogenes* (Group A, B or C), which produces an exotoxin.
Method of transmission:	Direct or intimate contact with a patient or carrier. Droplets from nasal carriers, that dry out and are carried by air currents are implicated in the spread of streptococci. They cling to dust, lint from bed linen, paper tissues, handkerchiefs or used towels, as well as to furniture and environmental structures. Ingestion of contaminated food such as eggs, milk and dairy products may also cause infection.
Incubation period:	Usually short, no longer than 1–3 days.
Infectious period:	10–21 days for treated, uncomplicated cases. If suppuration and sepsis is present, the secretions remain infectious far longer. If appropriate antibiotics are administered, the contagion ends within 24–48 hours. Within 2–3 weeks after exposure, untreated carriers gradually shed less streptococci, but they may remain carriers for longer.

CONTROL/PREVENTATIVE MEASURES						
Barrier measures		**Protective clothing**		**Housekeeping**		
Hand washing	✓	Gloves	✓	Cleaning		R
Hand disinfection	✓	Masks		Medical waste		R
Single room	✓	Caps		Laundry		R
Private room + b/room		Eye protection				
Separate equipment	✓	Cotton gowns				
Limit visitors	✓	Plastic aprons	✓			

Legal notification		**Readily communicable in the healthcare setting**	
On suspicion of infection		Yes	
On lab confirmation		No	✓

R = Routine   S = Special

Comments: Type-specific immunity develops after exposure to one of the streptococcal infections, even if no overt clinical symptoms were present. Trans-placental passive immunity is present in the newborn, but only to the type-specific antibodies the mother was exposed to. The toxin of another of the three groups of streptococci may trigger a second attack of scarlet fever. Administering antibiotics may interfere with the development of long-term type-specific immunity.

ICD-10- J12   SEVERE ACUTE RESPIRATORY SYNDROME
(SARS-CoV, SARS)

Signs and symptoms:	Acute pyrexia (>38°C), chills, rigor, myalgia, headache, diarrhoea, pharyngitis, rhinorrhoea, anorexia, skin rash, confusion, cough, shortness of breath, difficulty in breathing, pneumonia, acute respiratory distress syndrome (severe cases present with critical respiratory illness, requiring oxygen support and/or mechanical ventilation. X-rays may or may not show chest abnormalities).
Causative organism:	A virus: SARS-associated coronavirus (SARS-CoV)
Method of transmission:	Contact with respiratory secretions (aerosol and droplet spread) and faeces.
Incubation period:	3–7 days, sometimes as long as 10 days.
Infectious period:	As long as viable virus is present in secretions and faeces. Research has shown that a viable virus can be cultured from environmental surfaces for as long as 24 hours after exposure. Diarrhoea may remain infective even longer, as the virus is protected well by the stool.

CONTROL/PREVENTATIVE MEASURES					
Barrier measures		**Protective clothing**		**Housekeeping**	
Hand washing	✓	Gloves	✓	Cleaning	S
Hand disinfection	✓	Masks	✓	Medical waste	R
Single room		Caps	✓	Laundry	S
Private room + b/room	✓	Eye protection	✓		
Separate equipment	✓	Cotton gowns			
Limit visitors	✓	Plastic aprons	✓		

Legal notification		**Readily communicable in the healthcare setting**	
On suspicion of infection		Yes	✓
On lab confirmation		No	

R = Routine   S = Special

Comments: Healthcare workers exposed to the secretions of infected patients are at risk of contracting SARS. Epidemiologic criteria for possible SARS-CoV diagnosis include:

- Any signs and symptoms of infection, combined with a history of travel to a domestic or foreign suspected/confirmed epidemic/endemic area within 10 days of onset of illness.
- Close contact* with a person with moderate to severe respiratory illness and a possible exposing travel history within the previous 10 days before onset of symptoms.
- Close contact* with a person with confirmed SARS-CoV infection.
- Close contact* with a person with mild, moderate or severe respiratory illness, where a chain of transmission can be linked to a confirmed case of SARS-CoV disease within the 10 days before the onset of symptoms.

Close contact is defined as face-to-face contact, or contact with body fluids from patients with suspected or confirmed SARS.

The Center for Disease Control and Prevention (CDC), in Atlanta, Georgia, USA has suggested specific community containment measures as detailed in the table below, including non-hospital isolation and quarantine for SARS contacts.

MONITORING OPTIONS	METHOD
1. Passive monitoring ■ Low risk of infection or ■ Poor availability of resources or ■ The risk of delayed recognition of symptoms is low.	Contacts are placed under home quarantine, where they are required to do self-assessment at least twice daily and to contact the healthcare authorities immediately if respiratory symptoms or fever occurs.
2. Active monitoring without explicit activity restrictions ■ Moderate to high risk or ■ Resources permit close observation of contacts ■ The risk of delayed recognition of symptoms is moderate to high.	A healthcare worker evaluates the contact regularly, (at least daily) by telephone and/or in person, for signs and symptoms of possible SARS-CoV infection.
3. Active monitoring with activity restrictions (quarantine, e.g. voluntary or mandatory at home).	Law enforcement may be necessary to assist with the management of noncompliant persons.
4. Working quarantine (for persons for whom activity restrictions are indicated, but who provide essential services, such as healthcare workers).	The contact remains separated from others for at least 10 days after potential exposure and is assessed at least daily in person for signs and symptoms of possible SARS-CoV infection. May share with the household as long as the person remains asymptomatic. Minimise interaction with household members as far as possible during this period.
5. Focused measures to increase social distance.	Contacts are allowed to work, but must observe activity restrictions while off duty. Monitoring for fever and other symptoms before reporting for work, and using appropriate personal protective equipment such as N95 high-particulate filter masks, are required.
6. Community-wide measures to increase social distance, used for protection of all members of a community where ■ Extensive transmission of SARS-CoV is occurring or ■ A significant number of cases lack clearly identifiable epidemiological links ■ Restrictions on known exposed persons are considered insufficient to prevent further spread.	Monitoring specific groups in order to reduce interactions and transmission risk, e.g. workers in specific sites or buildings, where most, but not necessarily all, persons are at risk of exposure. Typically includes closure of schools, workplaces, public buildings and mass transport, cancellation of large events or meetings.

MONITORING OPTIONS	METHOD
7. Widespread community quarantine, including cordon sanitaire (sanitary barrier), for protection of all the members of a community, housing complex or office building, where ■ Extensive transmission of SARS-CoV is occurring or ■ A significant number of cases lack clearly identifiable epidemiological links. Restrictions on known exposed persons are considered insufficient to prevent further spread.	Legal enforcement restricting movement into or out of an area of quarantine of a large group of people, designed to reduce the risk of transmission of SARS-CoV among persons in, and to persons outside, the affected area. Law enforcement may be necessary to assist with the management of noncompliant persons.

ICD-10- A03   SHIGELLOSIS *(Bacillary dysentry)*

Signs and symptoms: An acute disease of the large and distal small intestine, characterised by diarrhoea, fever, nausea, sometimes toxaemia, vomiting, cramps and tenesmus. Stools contain blood, mucus and pus (dysentery) from the micro-abscesses caused by the micro-organisms in the enteric mucosa. About one third of sufferers present with watery diarrhoea. Convulsions may occur in children. Asymptomatic to mild cases are common. The disease is usually self-limiting and seldom lasts more than 4–7 days. The severity of the attack is determined by the nutrition and age of the patient (very young or elderly) and the serotype of the infecting organism. A mortality rate of 5–10% is common among the very young or elderly.

Causative organism: A bacterium – *Shigella.* Group A = *S. dysenteriae*; Group B = *S. flexneri*; Group C = *S. boydii*; Group D = *S. sonnei*; – each with different sero- and subtypes.

Method of transmission: Direct and indirect faecal-oral transmission from a patient or carrier. Ingestion of contaminated food (especially milk products) and water is often implicated. Flies contaminate unrefrigerated food, causing the bacteria to multiply until sufficient numbers for an infectious dose are achieved. Very few (10–100) organisms are needed for an infecting dose.

Incubation period: 12–96 hours, on average 1–3 days (or even a week for *S. dysenteriae* 1).

Infectious period: During the stage of acute infection until the organism is no longer present in the stool (+/-4 weeks). Asymptomatic carriers may transmit the infection for many months. Appropriate antibiotic treatment usually reduces the infectious carrier stage to less than a week.

CONTROL/PREVENTATIVE MEASURES

Barrier measures		Protective clothing		Housekeeping	
Hand washing	✓	Gloves	✓	Cleaning	S
Hand disinfection	✓	Masks		Medical waste	R
Single room		Caps		Laundry	R
Private room + b/room	✓	Eye protection			
Separate equipment	✓	Cotton gowns			
Limit visitors	✓	Plastic aprons	✓		

Legal notification		Readily communicable in the healthcare setting	
On suspicion of infection		Yes	✓
On lab confirmation		No	

R = Routine   S = Special

Comments: Overcrowding and poor sanitation promote the outbreak of shigellosis. Healthcare facilities (crèches, hospitals and day-care centers) and institutions such as prisons are high-risk areas for outbreaks of diarrhoea. Contacts and infected patients and/or carriers may not handle children, food or patients before 2 consecutive negative stool specimens, collected 24 hours apart and 48 hours from when the last dose of antibiotic was administered, indicate that they are no longer infectious. The specimens must be sent to the microbiology laboratory for culturing. Debilitated patients should be evaluated for signs of dehydration, which may be fatal in severe cases. Education regarding personal hygiene to combat the spread of the infection is important for both the patient and family.

ICD-10-B03   SMALLPOX *(Variola)*

Signs and symptoms:	An extremely infectious disease with a sudden onset, fever, malaise, headache, severe backache, prostration and occasionally abdominal pain. After 2–4 days the temperature drops and a rash appears, which passes through successive stages of macules, papules, vesicles, pustules and finally scabs. The fever frequently intensifies as the rash progresses to the pustular stage. The lesions are more abundant on the face and limbs. The disease persists for 3–4 weeks. Haemorrhagic symptoms usually accompany fatal infections.
Causative organism:	A virus: variola virus.
Method of transmission:	Close contact with respiratory discharges (nasal and pharyngeal); drainage from vesicles or skin lesions; contaminated clothing/bed linen.
Incubation period:	7–17 days. The symptoms become apparent within 10–12 days and the rash appears 2–4 days later.
Infectious period:	From a few days before the development of the earliest symptoms (rash) until the last scabs have disappeared in +/-3 weeks. Most communicable during the first week.

CONTROL/PREVENTATIVE MEASURES

Barrier measures		Protective clothing		Housekeeping	
Hand washing	✓	Gloves	✓	Cleaning	S
Hand disinfection	✓	Masks (95% high particulate filter type)		Medical waste	R
Single room		Caps	✓	Laundry	R
Private room + b/room	✓	Eye protection			
Separate equipment	✓	Cotton gowns			
Limit visitors	✓	Plastic aprons	✓		

Legal notification		Readily communicable in the healthcare setting	
On suspicion of infection		Yes	✓
On lab confirmation	✓	No	

R = Routine   S = Special

Comments: No specific treatment is available against smallpox. Patients should preferably be admitted to a Priority 4 isolation unit where special isolation facilities and staff are available. An effective vaccine is available, although many countries have stopped vaccinating their populations. According to the World Health Organization, smallpox has been eradicated world-wide since 1980. Household, work or school contacts are especially exposed to variola. Laundry staff handling contaminated linen are considered to be at special risk as well. All materials and items which have come into contact with the patient have to be pasteurised (by boiling), steam autoclaved or incinerated. Tracing and examining contacts is of the utmost importance. Work/school exclusion extends until the attending doctor certifies full recovery and all scabs have dropped off. Smallpox is a pathogen often associated with a possible bioterrorism threat.

ICD-10-A50 to A52   SYPHILIS *(Chancre, lues)*

Signs and symptoms: A contagious venereal disease, characterised by acute active manifestations and periods of latency in untreated cases.

Three stages are described:

Primary syphilis: A primary lesion (chancre) appears about 3 weeks after exposure as a painless ulcer with a serous exudate on the site of the initial invasion (e.g. the genitalia). In women it may be internal and unnoticed, or appear on the lips, eyelids or anus. The ulcer disappears after 10–14 days, even without treatment. Ulcers may recur. A firm, painless satellite lymph node (bubo) commonly develops.

Secondary syphilis (in untreated cases): Follows 2–6 months after the disappearance of the primary ulcer, may last as long as 2 years. The ulcers usually disappear spontaneously within 3–12 weeks. The disease is highly infectious at this stage. A symmetrical, copper-coloured rash, similar to measles, first appears on the soles and palms, spreading to the rest of the skin surface. White sores may appear on the mucosa of the mouth and throat, around the genitalia and rectum. Headache, fever and a general feeling of illness is common. Hair loss, aching joints and anaemia may develop, and the eyes may be affected.

Tertiary syphilis (late syphilis): Symptoms may develop soon after secondary syphilis or remain hidden for up to 15 years or longer. Blood tests may be negative and the person may be unaware that he/she has the disease. Late syphilis is less contagious, but extremely dangerous to the person who has it. Infectious granulomas (gummas) may develop in the skin, viscera, bones or mucosa. It can be fatal when the heart or central nervous system is affected. All internal organs, bones, joints and blood vessels may be affected and/or destroyed. Insanity, paresis or perforation of the soft palate may occur. Deep ulcera may appear on the limbs.

Causative organism: A bacterium (spirochete): *Treponema pallidum.*

Method of transmission: By direct contact with infectious secretion from skin lesions or mucous membranes, or through sexual contact. Total infection occurs through placental transfer or at delivery.

Incubation period: 10 days–3 months, usually 3 weeks.

Infectious period: Difficult to determine. Adequate antibiotic treatment ends infectivity within 24–48 hours. Untreated syphilis may remain infectious for 2–4 years. In pregnant women transmission to the foetus will most likely take place during the primary stage, or during the latent period of infection.

CONTROL/PREVENTATIVE MEASURES

Barrier measures		Protective clothing		Housekeeping	
Hand washing	✓	Gloves	✓	Cleaning	R
Hand disinfection	✓	Masks (during delivery)	✓	Medical waste	R
Single room		Caps (during delivery)	✓	Laundry	R
Private room + b/room		Eye protection (during delivery)	✓		
Separate equipment	✓	Cotton gowns			
Limit visitors		Plastic aprons	✓		

Legal notification		Readily communicable in the healthcare setting	
On suspicion of infection		Yes	
On lab confirmation of congenital syphilis	✓	No	✓

R = Routine   S = Special

Comments: Healthcare workers must wear appropriate protective clothing while performing any procedure on an infected patient. Infection with syphilis does not provide immunity and the treated person may be reinfected. Congenital syphilis is a legally notifiable disease. Eye protection against splatters of amniotic fluid or blood is advisable in the labour ward. No sexual contact is advisable while there is drainage from skin lesions. Screening of all sexual contacts and treatment, when necessary, is important. No school or work exclusion is necessary.

ICD-10-B68   TAENIASIS *(Tapeworm, pork and beef tapeworm)*

Signs and symptoms:	Nervousness, insomnia, anorexia, loss of weight, abdominal pain and digestive disturbances (e.g. obstruction and rectal itching). Segments of tapeworm and its eggs are passed anally. Infestation is usually not fatal and may continue asymptomatically for years. Human hosts usually harbour only one tapeworm at a time.
Causative organism:	A worm (nematode): *Taenia solium* (pork tapeworm) or *Taenia saginata* (beef tapeworm).
Method of transmission:	Ingestion of contaminated raw or half-cooked pork or beef. Faecal-oral transmission readily takes place if the hands are contaminated with eggs, as may happen with children, the mentally handicapped or food handlers.
Incubation period:	Within 8–14 weeks eggs appear in the stools of infested persons.
Infectious period:	Pork tapeworm is directly transmitted from person-to-person; beef tapeworm is not. As long as the worm lives in the intestine it will lay eggs that are passed by the human host. The eggs remain viable in the environment for months. An adult worm may live up to 30 years.

CONTROL/PREVENTATIVE MEASURES

Barrier measures		Protective clothing		Housekeeping	
Hand washing	✓	Gloves	✓	Cleaning	R
Hand disinfection	✓	Masks		Medical waste	R
Single room		Caps		Laundry	R
Private room + b/room		Eye protection			
Separate equipment		Cotton gowns			
Limit visitors		Plastic aprons	✓		

Legal notification		Readily communicable in the healthcare setting	
On suspicion of infection		Yes	
On lab confirmation		No	✓

R = Routine   S = Special

Comments: Freezing and keeping pork and beef at a temperature below -5°C (23°F) for more than 4 days kills the cysts. Thorough inspection of all meat before human consumption is necessary. Reinfection of a recovered person is common. Poor sanitation and hand hygiene contributes to the problem. Ensuring good hand hygiene at all times generally prevents infestation. Cysticercosis, a larval infection, is a serious disease that may involve many different body organs. When eggs of the pork tapeworm are swallowed, they hatch in the small intestine. The larvae migrate to the subcutaneous tissue, striated muscle or other vital organs and form cysts (the cysticerci). If the cysts localise in the patient's heart, eyes or brain and/or central nervous system, the consequences may be grave. Neuro-cysticercosis may cause serious disability and carries a high fatality rate. Its symptoms can appear within days to 10 years after infection.

ICD-10-A33-5   TETANUS *(Lockjaw, tetanus neonatorum)*

Signs and symptoms:	An acute **intoxication**, characterised by painful muscular contractions of the jaw, an inability to swallow, stiffness of the neck, fever, headache, restlessness and convulsions. Usually has a poor prognosis and a high mortality rate (30–90%). The muscles of the face, neck and abdomen may spasm. In severe cases, a loud noise or sudden movement may cause convulsions. With *Tetanus neonatorum*, the symptoms usually occur during days 5–12 after birth. If the disease develops soon after exposure, the prognosis is poor and the symptoms more severe.
Causative organism:	The toxin, from the bacterium: *Clostridium tetani.*
Method of transmission:	Tetanus spores are present in soil, dust, and human and animal faeces. The spores are introduced into the body during injury, especially lacerations, traumatic abrasions and burns contaminated with soil, which carry a high risk of infection. *Tetanus neonatorum* usually occurs due to infection of the unhealed umbilicus, particularly if the umbilical cord is 'treated' with poultices of animal dung. Intravenous drug users may spread the infection by sharing contaminated syringes and needles.
Incubation period:	3–21 days, average 10–14 days. In neonates, the incubation period is 3–28 days, with an average of 6 days.
Infectious period:	Not directly transmitted from person-to-person.

CONTROL/PREVENTATIVE MEASURES

Barrier measures		Protective clothing		Housekeeping	
Hand washing	✓	Gloves	✓	Cleaning	R
Hand disinfection	✓	Masks		Medical waste	R
Single room	✓	Caps		Laundry	R
Private room + b/room		Eye protection			
Separate equipment		Cotton gowns			
Limit visitors	✓	Plastic aprons	✓		

Legal notification		Readily communicable in the healthcare setting	
On suspicion of infection		Yes	
On lab confirmation	✓	No	✓

R = Routine   S = Special

Comments: Active immunisation is available (antitoxin and toxoid) which protects the recipient for 3–10 years. Booster doses should be given every 5-10 years. Immunisation during early pregnancy is preferable to protect the fetus. All patients with tetanus must be hospitalised. The infected patient is treated symptomatically. The penetration wound may need to be surgically dissected and toxoid injected into the tissues around it. Because the bacteria can grow anaerobically, all necrotic tissue should be removed as soon as possible. The environment should be kept as quiet as possible. Mother/child education as well as maternity care in rural areas needs to improve to combat (potentially) dangerous ethnic and cultural practices.

ICD-10-A77   TICK BITE FEVER *(Tick fever, rickettsiosis, spotted fever)*

Signs and symptoms:	A sudden onset with a moderate to high fever lasting 2–3 weeks in untreated cases. Symptoms include extreme exhaustion, malaise, deep muscle pain, severe headache, chills and conjunctivitis. From about the third day a maculopapular rash develops on the limbs, spreading to the palms of the hands and soles of the feet. The rash rapidly spreads to most of the body. Petechiae and subcutaneous haemorrhages are common. A necrotic area surrounded by cellulitis forms at the site of the bite, while the surrounding lymph glands enlarge.
Causative organism:	A rickettsia: *Rickettsiae pijperi* or *R. rickettsii*.
Method of transmission:	The bite of an infected tick. The infection may also be caused by contamination of the host's skin or the bite wound with tissue from the crushed tick, or its faeces.
Incubation period:	Usually 3–14 days, average 7 days.
Infectious period:	Not directly transmitted from person-to-person. The tick remains infective throughout its life span, surviving for as long as 18 months under very favourable conditions.

CONTROL/PREVENTATIVE MEASURES					
Barrier measures		**Protective clothing**		**Housekeeping**	
Hand washing	✓	Gloves	✓	Cleaning	R
Hand disinfection	✓	Masks		Medical waste	R
Single room		Caps		Laundry	R
Private room + b/room		Eye protection			
Separate equipment		Cotton gowns			
Limit visitors		Plastic aprons	✓		

Legal notification		**Readily communicable in the healthcare setting**	
On suspicion of infection		Yes	
On lab confirmation		No	✓

R = Routine   S = Special

Comments: Rickettsiae are activated and become infective within hours after the tick has had its first meal of blood. Active immunity probably lasts for years. Pets, goats, sheep and cattle may carry and spread ticks. The patient's contacts must be monitored and where exposure has taken place, treated according to their symptoms. No school or work exclusion is necessary, unless the patient's condition requires it.

ICD-10-B58   TOXOPLASMOSIS

Signs and symptoms: A systemic infection, often asymptomatic. Fever, lymphadenopathy and lymphocytosis may persist for days or weeks. As soon as antibodies develop, the parasitaemia decreases. The toxoplasma cysts remaining in the tissues contain viable parasites even when the parasitaemia decreases. In immunodeficient patients the symptoms include cerebral and eye anomalies, pneumonia, general skeletal and muscular impairment, myocarditis, a red maculopapular rash, coma and death. A primary infection during early pregnancy may lead to intrauterine death or foetal abnormalities. Cerebral toxoplasmosis often accompanies HIV infection.

Causative organism: A protozoa: *Toxoplasma gondii* (found worldwide in cats, other mammals and birds).

Method of transmission: Transplacental transmission during early pregnancy. Children coming into contact with contaminated soil in sandpits, gardens and play areas. Ingestion of contaminated, under-cooked meat, water or food. Rarely, organ transplants or blood transfusion from an infected donor.

Incubation period: 10–23 days after ingestion of contaminated food.
5–20 days after contact with infectious animals, especially cats.

Infectious period: Not directly transmitted from person-to-person, except transplacentally. Contaminated water or moist soil may remain infective for as long as a year. Cysts in contaminated meat remain infectious as long as the meat is uncooked, but edible.

CONTROL/PREVENTATIVE MEASURES					
Barrier measures		**Protective clothing**		**Housekeeping**	
Hand washing	✓	Gloves	✓	Cleaning	R
Hand disinfection	✓	Masks		Medical waste	R
Single room		Caps		Laundry	R
Private room + b/room		Eye protection			
Separate equipment		Cotton gowns			
Limit visitors		Plastic aprons			

Legal notification		Readily communicable in the healthcare setting	
On suspicion of infection		Yes	
On lab confirmation		No	✓

R = Routine   S = Special

Comments: No immunisation is available. Meat must always be well cooked, until it changes colour to the bone. Freezing meat reduces but does not eliminate the infectiveness of the organism. The hygiene of pets, especially cats and their litterbins, must be checked regularly. Gardeners should wear gloves, especially if pets roam the area. Washing hands with care after handling cats and birds/birdcages is a good precaution against infection.

ICD-10-A71   TRACHOMA

Signs and symptoms:	An infectious conjunctivitis with an insidious or abrupt onset and a purulent conjunctival exudate, which may persist for years in untreated patients, characterised by frequent reinfection. Severe pain and superficial vascularisation of the cornea is common. Ulceration of the cornea leads to progressive scarring and even blindness in untreated patients. Scarring of the conjunctiva causes turned-in eyelids and eyelid deformities. This may worsen the corneal abrasion, leading to visual impairment.
Causative organism:	A specialised bacterium: *Chlamydia trachomatis,* an organism with some characteristics of Gram-negative bacteria, functioning as an intracellular parasite.
Method of transmission:	Direct contact with ocular discharges of infected patients. Possibly caused by contact with purulent nasopharyngeal drainage as well. Flies and contaminated clothing, towels and other personal possessions may spread the infection.
Incubation period:	5–12 days.
Infectious period:	As long as the organism is present in the conjunctiva, mucous membrane lesions and ocular exudate. Contagion is terminated within 2–3 days of appropriate antibiotic treatment, although the clinical signs may still persist for a period of time.

CONTROL/PREVENTATIVE MEASURES					
Barrier measures		**Protective clothing**		**Housekeeping**	
Hand washing	✓	Gloves	✓	Cleaning	R
Hand disinfection	✓	Masks		Medical waste	R
Single room		Caps		Laundry	S
Private room + b/room		Eye protection			
Separate equipment	✓	Cotton gowns			
Limit visitors	✓	Plastic aprons	✓		

Legal notification		**Readily communicable in the healthcare setting**	
On suspicion of infection		Yes	
On lab confirmation	✓	No	✓

R = Routine   S = Special

Comments: This micro-organism causes venereal disease as well. Treatment includes antibiotic therapy as well as plastic surgery to rectify scarring. Poor hygiene and overcrowding increases the spread of trachoma. Reinfection of cured persons is common.

ICD-10-A15 to A19   TUBERCULOSIS *(TB, consumption)*

Signs and symptoms:	A communicable, infectious and inflammatory disease that usually attacks the lungs, but may occur in any other part of the body as well. In adults, the early symptoms include listlessness, loss of weight and vague chest pain that may pass unnoticed. Late in the course of the illness: night sweat, fever, cough, chest pain, hoarseness, purulent secretions and haemoptysis manifest. Pulmonary and extrapulmonary tuberculosis (miliary, meningeal and other less common types) are found.
Causative organism:	A bacterium: *Mycobacterium tuberculosis* and *M. africanum* (extrapulmonary).
Method of transmission:	Droplet spread from undiagnosed/confirmed infected persons during breathing, coughing, sneezing or singing (pulmonary or laryngeal tuberculosis). Close contact over extended periods, e.g. overcrowded living conditions, increases the incidence of transmission. Extrapulmonary tuberculosis (e.g. miliary) is less contagious than pulmonary tuberculosis, even in the presence of draining sinuses. Some experts maintain that powdered (dry) bacilli in dust pose a far greater risk than droplet spread.
Incubation period:	4–12 weeks. The latent infection may remain dormant for years.
Infectious period:	Theoretically as long as the bacilli are excreted in the sputum. 80% of untreated patients die within 2 years. HIV-positive tuberculosis patients may not respond to treatment as expected and should be considered infectious until clinically symptom-free.

CONTROL/PREVENTATIVE MEASURES FOR CASES WITH **DRUG SENSITIVE TUBERCULOSIS**

Barrier measures		Protective clothing		Housekeeping	
Hand washing	✓	Gloves	✓	Cleaning (especially droplet and dust control)	S
Hand disinfection	✓	Masks (surgical)	✓	Medical waste	R
Single room (at least the first 7 days)	✓	Caps		Laundry	R
Private room + b/room		Eye protection			
Separate equipment (at least the first 7 days)	✓	Cotton gowns			
Limit visitors (at least the first 7 days)	✓	Plastic aprons	✓		

Legal notification		Possibly communicable in the healthcare setting	
On suspicion of infection		Yes	✓
On lab confirmation	✓	No	

R = Routine   S = Special

CONTROL/PREVENTATIVE MEASURES FOR CASES WITH **MULTI-DRUG-RESISTANT TUBERCULOSIS (MDR TB)**

Barrier measures		Protective clothing		Housekeeping	
Hand washing	✓	Gloves	✓	Cleaning (especially droplet and dust control)	R
Hand disinfection	✓	Masks (95% high particulate filter type mask)	✓	Medical waste	R
Single room		Caps		Laundry	R
Private room + b/room		Eye protection			
Separate equipment	✓	Cotton gowns			
Limit visitors	✓	Plastic aprons	✓		

Legal notification		Readily communicable in the healthcare setting	
On suspicion of infection		Yes	✓
On lab confirmation	✓	No	

R = Routine   S = Special

Comments: Staff must wear masks while the patient is infectious and presents with copious secretions. If the tuberculosis patient is HIV-positive, masks must be worn throughout hospitalisation. Microscopic culturing and sensitivity tests are important in determining the appropriate treatment schedule for the patient. Unfortunately some test results take up to 6 weeks before they are available. Meanwhile treatment must be initiated in order to terminate infectivity as speedily as possible. Because most adults have been in contact with tuberculosis bacilli on a regular basis, tuberculin skin test results do not always reflect the true status of the person. HIV-positive persons are more susceptible to tuberculosis. Multi-drug-resistant tuberculosis is becoming a problem in southern Africa, especially in rural areas where diagnostic facilities are not readily available. Tracing the patient's intimate (household) contacts is very important. The exact treatment of the contacts depends on the individual and the circumstances. Directly observed treatment (DOTs) is the only really effective treatment option for containing the developing TB epidemic.

ICD-10-A01   TYPHOID FEVER *(Enteric fever)*

Signs and symptoms:	A systemic disease characterised by sustained fever, headache, malaise, anorexia, bradycardia, splenomegaly, a spotty rose-coloured rash on the trunk, a non-productive cough, and constipation more commonly than diarrhoea in adults. Intestinal perforation or haemorrhaging may occur in some untreated patients.
Causative organism:	A bacterium: *Salmonella typhii* (the typhoid bacillus).
Method of transmission:	Faecal-oral route, through contaminated food, milk and dairy products, fruit, vegetables and water. The organism is found in the faeces, urine or gallbladder of a patient/carrier. Flies spread the disease as well by infecting food.
Incubation period:	Usually 1–3 weeks, depending on the size of the infecting dose.
Infectious period:	As long as the typhoid bacillus is present in the secretions, usually from the first week until the convalescent period. In +/-10% of untreated cases bacilli are excreted for three months from the onset of the infection. 2–5% of patients become permanent carriers.

CONTROL/PREVENTATIVE MEASURES

Barrier measures		Protective clothing		Housekeeping	
Hand washing	✓	Gloves	✓	Cleaning	R
Hand disinfection	✓	Masks		Medical waste	R
Single room		Caps		Laundry	R
Private room + b/room	✓	Eye protection			
Separate equipment	✓	Cotton gowns			
Limit visitors	✓	Plastic aprons	✓		

Legal notification		Readily communicable in the healthcare setting	
On suspicion of infection		Yes	✓
On lab confirmation	✓	No	

R = Routine   S = Special

Comments: The public must be educated to wash their hands before meals and after bowel movements. Proper personal hygiene and the use of paper towels to prevent recontamination of the hands after defecating is important. The control of flies is in the public interest. Food, water and milk should always be pasteurised or boiled. Water can be chlorinated by adding 20 ml of household bleach to 25 litres of filtered water. Typhoid carriers should not handle food commercially. Immunisation against typhoid is available. Work/school exclusion is indicated until the course of treatment has been completed and at least three consecutive negative stool/urine specimens (depending on the source of the patient's infection) have been cultured. The specimens are to be collected at least 24 hours apart and 48 hours after the completion of the course of antibiotics. The personal contacts of both typhoid and paratyphoid fever patients must be screened for infection.

ICD-10-A75.2   TYPHUS FEVER *(Flea-borne)*

Signs and symptoms:	Similar symptoms to those of louse-borne typhus, only milder. A seasonal distribution of the disease is characteristic and sporadic outbreaks during warm weather are common.
Causative organism:	A rickettsia: *Rickettsiae typhii (R. mooseri).*
Method of transmission:	Infected rat fleas excrete rickettsiae while feeding, contaminating the bite site in the process. Dried infected faeces may be inhaled in dust, causing infection.
Incubation period:	1–2 weeks, usually 12 days.
Infectious period:	Not directly transmitted from person-to-person. Fleas are infective for life and may live for as long as 12 months.

CONTROL/PREVENTATIVE MEASURES						
Barrier measures		**Protective clothing**		**Housekeeping**	
Hand washing	✓	Gloves	✓	Cleaning	R
Hand disinfection	✓	Masks		Medical waste	R
Single room		Caps		Laundry	R
Private room + b/room		Eye protection			
Separate equipment	✓	Cotton gowns			
Limit visitors		Plastic aprons	✓		

Legal notification		**Readily communicable in the healthcare setting**	
On suspicion of infection		Yes	
On lab confirmation	✓	No	✓

R = Routine   S = Special

Comments: After the patient, his/her clothes and the environment have been treated and are no longer infested, no further protective barriers are needed. Further treatment is symptomatic. Home quarantine is still advised in some areas: isolation is implemented for 15 days after surfaces have been treated with an appropriate contact/residual insecticide. Trace intimate contacts of the patient and observe for 2 weeks for early symptoms. The infection is common in areas of poor sanitation and overcrowding. The use of insect repellents and insecticides in endemic areas is indicated. One attack usually confers immunity.

ICD-10-A75.0   TYPHUS FEVER *(Louse-borne)*

Signs and symptoms:	Sudden onset with fever, headache, rigor, prostration and general pain. On the second to sixth day a macular rash appears on the body, excluding the face, palms of the hands and soles of the feet. Toxaemia is usually pronounced. The fever may last for 2 weeks. In the absence of specific treatment, the fatality rate may increase from between 10–40% with increase in the patient's age .
Causative organism:	A rickettsiae: *Rickettsiae prowazekii.*
Method of transmission:	The bite of an infected body-louse *Pediculus humanus corporis.* Carriers of typhus are a source of infection for the lice. Infection by inhalation of the faeces of the body louse in dust is possible. Abrasions and lacerations may be infected with lice faeces.
Incubation period:	1–2 weeks, usually 12 days.
Infectious period:	Not directly transmitted from person-to-person. Infected patients may infect lice during the febrile illness and 2–3 days after the temperature returns to normal. The lice pass rickettsiae in their faeces within 2–6 days after exposure. Lice usually die within +/-2 weeks but rickettsiae remain viable in the dead lice for weeks.

CONTROL/PREVENTATIVE MEASURES						
Barrier measures		**Protective clothing**		**Housekeeping**		
Hand washing	✓	Gloves	✓	Cleaning		R
Hand disinfection	✓	Masks		Medical waste		R
Single room		Caps		Laundry		R
Private room + b/room		Eye protection				
Separate equipment	✓	Cotton gowns				
Limit visitors	✓	Plastic aprons	✓			

Legal notification		**Readily communicable in the healthcare setting**	
On suspicion of infection		Yes	
On lab confirmation	✓	No	✓

R = Routine   S = Special

Comments: After the patient, his/her clothes and the environment have been deloused, no further protective barriers are needed. Further treatment is symptomatic. The patient's hair must be examined and treated if any nits are seen. Home quarantine is still advised in some areas: isolation is implemented for 15 days after surfaces have been treated with an appropriate contact/residual insecticide. Trace intimate contacts of the patient and observe for 2 weeks for early symptoms. The infection is common in areas of poor sanitation and overcrowding. The use of insect repellents and insecticides in endemic areas is indicated. One attack usually confers immunity.

ICD-10-A98.0   VIRAL HAEMORRHAGIC FEVER: CRIMEAN-CONGO FEVER

Signs and symptoms:	Sudden onset of severe, persistent fever, malaise, weakness, anorexia, severe pain in limbs and abdomen. Erythema of face and chest, haemorrhagic enanthema of soft palate, uvula and pharynx. A petechial rash develops, spreading from the chest and abdomen to the rest of the body, forming large purpuric areas. Active haemorrhages may occur in the lungs, uterus, bladder and all other mucous membranes. Suppression of platelet formation is characteristic. Severe haemorrhage of the brain may cause coma and death. Convalescence is prolonged.
Causative organism:	A virus: the Crimean-Congo haemorrhagic fever virus (genus *Nairovirus*).
Method of transmission:	The bite of an infected *Hyalomma* tick or contact with the blood of an infected patient or animal.
Incubation period:	Primary contact (e.g. the patient): 5–9 days. Secondary contacts (e.g. healthcare staff): 3–6 days.
Infectious period:	During active haemorrhage, until an unspecified time after death. The duration of the disease is approximately 21 days and recovery depends on the active development of antibodies by the patient's immune system.

CONTROL/PREVENTATIVE MEASURES					
Barrier measures		**Protective clothing**		**Housekeeping**	
Hand washing	✓	Gloves (double)	✓	Cleaning	S
Hand disinfection	✓	Masks (95% high particulate filter type)	✓	Medical waste	R
Single room		Caps	✓	Laundry	S
Private room + b/room	✓	Eye protection	✓		
Separate equipment	✓	Gowns (impermeable)	✓		
Limit visitors	✓	Plastic aprons	✓		

Legal notification		**Readily communicable in the healthcare setting**	
On suspicion of infection	✓	Yes	✓
On lab confirmation	✓	No	

R = Routine   S = Special

Comments: A serious viral haemorrhagic disease that requires intensive and strict isolation and specific barrier nursing. Contacts must be located and monitored. A high-security isolation ward (e.g. P4 isolation) should be used to isolate suspected/confirmed cases. No treatment against the virus is available at present. Only symptomatic treatment is available (pyrexial and pain relief, plasma, blood and platelet transfusions). An attack confers lifelong immunity.

ICD-10-A63-B07	**WARTS** *(Venereal warts, condylomata acuminata, condylomata, papilloma venereum)*

Signs and symptoms:	Cauliflower-like, fleshy growths most often seen in moist areas in and around the genitalia and anus/anal canal. Genital warts are often associated with HIV-infection and may become malignant.
Causative organism:	A virus: the human papilloma virus.
Method of transmission:	Usually by direct contact with the lesions. Sexual transmission is common. Infection of the newborn may take place during vaginal delivery and manifest later with respiratory complications.
Incubation period:	1–20 months, average 2–3 months.
Infectious period:	Unknown, possibly as long as visible lesions persist. Immune-compromised persons are especially susceptible. The incidence in these persons increases as their immunity decreases.

CONTROL/PREVENTATIVE MEASURES

Barrier measures		Protective clothing		Housekeeping	
Hand washing	✓	Gloves	✓	Cleaning	R
Hand disinfection	✓	Masks		Medical waste	R
Single room		Caps		Laundry	R
Private room + b/room		Eye protection			
Separate equipment	✓	Cotton gowns			
Limit visitors		Plastic aprons	✓		

Legal notification		Readily communicable in the healthcare setting	
On suspicion of infection		Yes	
On lab confirmation		No	✓

R = Routine   S = Special

Comments: Within a few months to years, warts usually regress spontaneously but may flare up again unexpectedly. Surgery is necessary when warts obstruct the birth canal. Caesarean section should always be considered in severe cases of vaginal warts. Patients and their sexual partners should be educated about the need for good personal hygiene and infection control measures, including condom use.

ICD-10-A95   YELLOW FEVER

Signs and symptoms:	An acute infectious disease with sudden onset, fever, headache, back-ache, chills, prostration, nausea, vomiting, generalised muscle pain, bradycardia, progressive jaundice, weak pulse and haemorrhaging (e.g. haematemesis, epistaxis, melaena). The pulse is slow and weak, out of proportion to the pyrexia (Faget sign). Symptoms may vary from asymptomatic or mild, to fatal. 20–50% of jaundiced cases are fatal.
Causative organism:	A virus: yellow fever virus (*Flavivirus*).
Method of transmission:	The bite of an infected *Aedes aegypti* mosquito. Person-to-person transmission is possible due to transfusion or contact with infected blood.
Incubation period:	3–6 days.
Infectious period:	The patient's blood is infective for 3–5 days, starting shortly before commencement of the fever. The infection is not transferable through direct contact or fomites. Mosquitoes are infected for the duration of their life.

CONTROL/PREVENTATIVE MEASURES

Barrier measures		Protective clothing		Housekeeping	
Hand washing	✓	Gloves	✓	Cleaning	R
Hand disinfection	✓	Masks		Medical waste	R
Single room		Caps		Laundry	R
Private room + b/room		Eye protection			
Separate equipment	✓	Cotton gowns			
Limit visitors		Plastic aprons	✓		

Legal notification		Readily communicable in the healthcare setting	
On suspicion of infection		Yes	
On lab confirmation	✓	No	✓

R = Routine   S = Special

Comments: A vaccine is available. Lifelong immunity follows active infection. Certain international destinations require that travellers from Africa produce a current yellow fever vaccination certificate. Vaccination is possible at specialised travel clinics. Revaccination every 10 years is internationally accepted. Eradication of mosquitoes as a community project is indicated in endemic areas.

Fig.1: An example of Form GW 17/5

G.P.-S. 004-9045 | GW 17/5

Notification of medical condition
[Sections 32, 47 (i) (a) and 47 (i) (b) of Act No. 63 1977]
Department of Health

Aanmelding van mediese toestand
[Artikels 32, 47 (i) (a) en 47 (i) (b) van Wet No. 63 van 1977]
Departement van Gesondheid

Please print ● Where appropriate, mark the correct box with a tick (✓) ● Complete in duplicate. Original to be sent to local authority where patient was diagnosed: copy to remain in book.

Gebruik asseblief drukskrif ● Waar toepaslik, merk die korrekte blok (✓) ● Voltooi in duplikaat. Die oorspronklike word gestuur aan die plaaslike owerheid waar die pasiënt gediagnoseer is: die afskrif bly in die boek.

DETAILS OF PATIENT — BESONDERHEDE VAN PASIËNT

Surname ______ Van | First names ______ Voornaame

Age ______ Ouderdom | Sex: *Male* ☐ *Manlik* / *Female* ☐ *Vroulik* — Geslag | Ethnic group: *Asian* ☐ *Asiër* / *Black* ☐ *Swart* / *Coloured* ☐ *Kleurling* / *White* ☐ *Blank* — Etniese groep

Residential address .... Woonadres

If resident on a farm, state farmer's name as well as name and number of farm. In other rural areas, give name of chief, induna, village, nearest hill or river, nearest school or clinic .... Indien woonagtig op 'n plaas, noem die boer se naam sowel as die naam en nommer van die plaas. In ander landelike gebiede, gee die naam van die stamkaptein, induna, dorp, naaste heuwel of rivier, naaste skool of kliniek

District .... Distrik

Tel. No. .... Tel. No.

Name and address of employer, school, crèche or other institution where patient spends much of the day .... Naam en adres van werkgewer, skool, crèche of ander instelling waar die pasiënt 'n groot gedeelte van die dag is

Tel. No. .... Tel. No.

DETAILS OF MEDICAL CONDITION — BESONDERHEDE VAN MEDIESE TOESTAND

Medical condition ______ Mediese toestand

Date of onset ______ Aanvangsdatum | Date of death (if applicable) ______ Sterftedatum (indien van toepassing)

Possible place of infection ______ Moontlike plek van infeksie

Diagnosis was based on: *Clinical history and examination only* ☐ *Net kliniese geskiedenis en ondersoek* / *Clinical and other investigations* ☐ *Kliniese en ander ondersoeke* — Diagnose is gebaseer op

RESULTS OF INVESTIGATIONS — ONDERSOEKRESULTATE

Investigation (excluding TB sputum) ↓ Ondersoek (TB sputum uitgesluit)	Results ↓ Resultate
	Awaiting result ☐ *Wag vir resultate*
	Awaiting result ☐ *Wag vir resultate*
	Awaiting result ☐ *Wag vir resultate*

If TB, give sputum results ⟶ | Microscopy: *Positive* ☐ *Positief* / *Negative* ☐ *Negatief* / *Awaiting results* ☐ *Wag vir resultate* — Mikroskopie | Culture: *Positive* ☐ *Positief* / *Negative* ☐ *Negatief* / *Awaiting results* ☐ *Wag vir resultate* — Kultuur | ⟵ Indien TB, gee sputum resultate

REFERRED TO — VERWYS NA

Name of hospital or clinic ______ Naam van hospitaal of kliniek

Patient Registration No. ______ Pasiënt Registrasie No. | Date of administration ______ Datum van opname

NOTIFIED BY — AANGEMELD DEUR

Name ______ Naam

Address .... Adres | Profession: *Medical practitioner* ☐ *Geneesheer* / *Nurse* ☐ *Verpleegster* / *Other* ☐ *Ander* — Beroep

Signature ______ Handtekening

Tel. No. .... Tel. No. | Date ______ Datum

Local authority: If a copy of this notification is to be sent to another local authority, please confirm whether you will include this notification in your weekly summaries (GW 17/3 or 17/4). *Yes* ☐ *Ja* / *No* ☐ *Nee* *Plaaslike owerheid: Indien 'n afskrif van hierdie aanmelding aan 'n ander plaaslike owerheid gestuur word, bevestig asseblief of hierdie aanmelding by weeklikse opsomming (GW 17/3 of 17/4) ingesluit gaan word.*

REPLY BY LOCAL AUTHORITY — ANTWOORD DEUR PLAASLIKE OWERHEID

Reply to referring doctor/nurse with brief report of further findings and management. — Antwoord aan verwysende dokter/verpleegster oor verdere bevindinge en hantering.

Signature ______ Handtekening | Date ______ Datum | Tel. No. ______ Tel. No.

3 | Incident-related or hospital-acquired infections

General preventative and control measures

Incident-related or hospital-acquired infection is defined as clinical infection developing 48 hours or longer after hospitilisation, without any signs or symptoms of infection on admission.

Patients mainly develop hospital-acquired infections after undergoing penetrating procedures or after spending sufficient time in hospital to become colonised with or infected by micro-organisms from the environment. Most hospital environments harbour transient organisms from the patients, staff and visitors who have recently visited or worked in the area, as well as permanent micro-organisms that 'live' as hospital pathogens on furniture, in water systems, and on structures and equipment. Hospital pathogens usually have been in contact with anti-microbial agents, and they have developed genetically transmissable resistance to the most commonly used antibiotics. This resistance is transmitted from generation to generation. Some bacteria can multiply as quickly as every twenty minutes when a single bacterium divides in two, so many thousands of generations of resistant bacteria may develop within a day. These 'improved' species cause more severe and less treatable disease, resulting in a higher incidence of morbidity and mortality.

Healthcare staff must be sensitive to the possibility of hospital-acquired infections developing in patients and take the necessary precautions. Patients with a high risk of developing infection must be protected from admission. For example, persons older than 65 years and younger than 6 months of age are more prone to infection. Other groups include immunocompromised patients (e.g. those with underlying malignancy or immune suppression), patients with systemic metabolic disease, paralysis, lung pathology, extended trauma, post-anaesthesia and/or surgery patients, as well as patients on mechanical ventilation or chemotherapy such as steroids or cytotoxic drugs.

The implications of hospital-acquired infections include those for:
- The patient: an increase in morbidity, mortality, suffering and financial loss.
- The family: lower family morale and an increase in family disruption, workload and financial loss.

- The healthcare worker: an increase in the workload and ward disruption, with a lowering of staff morale.
- The hospital: financial loss and an increased burden on the existing facilities.

In the following discussion, a short overview will be given of the most common hospital-acquired infections, as well as the preventative and control procedures they require.

The aim of this section is to give the healthcare worker a general basis from which to start devising and implementing infection control measures when the initial signs and symptoms of infection in a patient are identified but before a diagnosis is confirmed. As soon as a specific or tentative diagnosis is made, the staff will refer to the disease-specific measures as set out in chapter 2.

CONTACT-TRANSMITTED INFECTION e.g. herpatic whitlow, Crimean Congo fever, impetigo, candidiasis

Definition:	Transmissable diseases are conditions which are usually spread directly from person-to-person through contact with body fluids or tissues or indirectly through contact with non-living surfaces (e.g. contaminated/soiled toys, instruments) or vectors (insects).
Method of transmission:	Opportunistic pathogens find temporary or permanent shelter by colonising and/or infiltrating the new host's body/tissues. Any possible type of infection may be transmitted in this manner, including airborne diseases (before the droplets dry out, settle and start flaking off).
	For further information, refer to the discussions on bacteraemia (page 121), airborne diseases (page 119), urinary tract infection (page 132) and wound infection (page 134).

CONTROL/PREVENTATIVE MEASURES					
Barrier measures		**Protective clothing**		**Housekeeping**	
Hand washing	✓	Gloves	✓	Cleaning	R
Hand disinfection	✓	Masks (aseptic procedures)	✓	Medical waste	R
Single room		Caps (aseptic procedures)	✓	Laundry	R
Private room + b/room		Eye protection			
Separate equipment	✓	Cotton gowns			
Limit visitors		Plastic aprons	✓		

Legal notification		**Readily communicable in the healthcare setting**	
On suspicion of infection		Yes	✓
On lab confirmation		No	

R = Routine   S = Special

AIRBORNE SPREAD e.g. *measles, varicella, rubella, diphtheria, whooping cough, meningococcal meningitis, parotitis, scarlet fever, pulmonary tuberculosis*

Definition:	The transmission of pathogens through inhalation, contamination/soiling of the airways, hands, clothes or body of the patient (or staff member), with droplets or dust containing micro-organisms.
Discussion:	Most of the airborne contagious diseases are childhood ailments. The exceptions include diseases such as pulmonary tuberculosis, which attack susceptible adults as well. Airborne infections spread readily between sick patients and staff members in hospitals, as droplets are secreted during respiration, and whilst talking and laughing. An unmasked person's hands will collect micro-organisms as he/she breathes over them. Pathogenic micro-organisms are dispersed along with the droplets shed by patients/staff members and cling to dust particles in the environment. The contaminating drops dry out, powder or splinter off and become part of the dust load or cling to surfaces such as curtains or work surfaces. A number of these micro-organisms are carried to the new host's nose, mouth, face or other susceptible portals where they find new areas in which to multiply. Many airborne diseases are viral. Antibiotics are therefore only administered to prevent the development of secondary bacterial infections. They are not effective in preventing or controlling the patient's viraemia. In order to inhibit the growth of viruses, the patient has to be infected and actively develop antibodies himself, or be passively immunised.
General signs and symptoms:	Any or all of the following: fever, chills, stiffness of the neck, swollen glands, sore throat, coryza, headache, malaise, excessive nasal secretions, coughing, bloodshot eyes, prostration, vomiting (often accompanied by diarrhoea in small children). **Viral infections:** A reddish, sometimes itchy rash is common with viral conditions, appearing days to weeks after exposure. The palms of the hands and soles of the feet can also have a blotched appearance. **Destructive lung conditions:** Bloodstained sputum is a serious symptom in respiratory diseases such as pulmonary tuberculosis.
Diagnosis:	The diagnosis is made on the patient's history as well as the clinical signs and symptoms. Blood analysis in a laboratory is often of little value as the patient is most contagious during the incubation period before symptoms appear. By the time the person is clinically ill, most of the viraemia/bacteraemia has usually subsided.
Complications:	**Rubella:** Pneumonia, abnormal babies born to mothers that contracted the disease during the first trimester of pregnancy. **Diphtheria:** Respiratory distress due to the development of a pseudo-membrane; toxin secreted by the pathogen may cause permanent eye,

ear, nerve, heart or renal damage.

Whooping cough: Pneumonia, haemorrhaging of the brain, eyes, skin or mucous membranes, convulsions, hernias due to coughing fits, coma and death, especially amongst frail or neglected toddlers of less than a year old.

Measles: Pneumonia, diarrhoea, encephalitis with brain damage.

Mumps: Inflammation of the ovaries, testes, pancreas or brain, deafness, sterility amongst post-pubescent persons.

Scarlet fever: Pneumonia; rheumatic fever and myocarditis is common.

CONTROL/PREVENTATIVE MEASURES					
Barrier measures		**Protective clothing**		**Housekeeping**	
Hand washing	✓	Gloves	✓	Cleaning	S
Hand disinfection	✓	Masks (productive coughing)	✓	Medical waste	R
Single room	✓	Caps		Laundry	R
Private room + b/room		Eye protection			
Separate equipment	✓	Cotton gowns			
Limit visitors	✓	Plastic aprons			
		(productive coughing)	✓		

Legal notification		Readily communicable in the healthcare setting	
On suspicion of infection		Yes	
On lab confirmation		No (if infection prevention is practiced)	✓

R = Routine   S = Special

BACTERAEMIA/SEPTICAEMIA

Though this infection is not transmissable from person-to-person, it is included in this section because it develops in healthcare settings, often after patient-care procedures.

Definition:	**Bacteraemia** indicates the presence/invasion/multiplication of bacteria in the blood of the patient.
	Septicaemia is the progression of the bacteraemia to a level where clinical signs and symptoms have developed and infection is diagnosed. Toxin(s) produced by certain bacteria, or secreted by the host's damaged tissues whilst the bacteria multiply, may cause septicaemia as well (e.g. toxic shock syndrome).
Discussion:	Bacteraemia is often the temporary result of surgery or invasive procedures such as heart catheterisation, lancing of abscesses or venesection. Colonisation of intravenous devices or indwelling urethral catheters may lead to bacteraemia as well. Intravenous devices or procedures are often associated with Gram-negative bacteraemia, due to contamination of the wound or bloodstream with the patient's own skin pathogens. The septicaemic patient's secretions/excretions and blood are treated as infectious, in keeping with basic infection control measures.
General signs and symptoms:	A high fluctuating fever is generally associated with septicaemia. Initially rigor and chills are common. Skin disorders such as petechiae, purpura, papules, pustules and vesicles as well as erythema develop. Gram-negative bacteraemia presents with a sudden onset, fever, rigor, nausea, vomiting, diarrhoea and prostration.
Diagnosis:	The presence of aerobic and anaerobic bacteria is only detectable by microbiological laboratory analysis. At least two simultaneous blood cultures are required to positively identify the micro-organisms and suggest antibiotic treatment. If a patient has already received antibiotics, the growth of cultures may be retarded, even though viable bacteria are present in the blood. The (aseptic) technique used to obtain blood culture samples also determines the accuracy of the laboratory results.
Complications:	Secondary meningeal infections; pericarditis; endocarditis; development of metastatic abscess; arthritis; septic shock or death may result from bacteraemia. Admission to a critical care unit with mechanical life support, intensive intravenous fluid therapy, systemic antibiotics and surgical abscess drainage when indicated may become necessary to prevent septic shock. Extended bacteraemia due to immune suppression, delayed diagnosis, inappropriate or inadequate antibiotic therapy, poor patient response or micro-organism resistance may be fatal.

CONTROL/PREVENTATIVE MEASURES

Barrier measures		Protective clothing		Housekeeping	
Hand washing	✓	Gloves	✓	Cleaning	R
Hand disinfection	✓	Masks		Medical waste	R
Single room		Caps		Laundry	R
Private room + b/room		Eye protection			
Separate equipment	✓	Cotton gowns			
Limit visitors	✓	Plastic aprons	✓		

Legal notification		Readily communicable in the healthcare setting	
On suspicion of infection		Yes	
On lab confirmation		No	✓

R = Routine   S = Special

INTRAVENOUS CANNULA-RELATED INFECTIONS
e.g. phlebitis, thrombophlebitis, cellulitis

Definition:	Development of a hospital-acquired infection due to contamination of the patient's bloodstream by an intravenous cannula, the entrance wound or infusion fluid.
Discussion:	Cannula-related infections are usually endemic (restricted to a single patient) whereas contaminated infusion fluid may cause an epidemic. This type of infection may present with or without pyrexia and bacteraemia.
	Phlebitis is usually the first sign of infection: the inflamed vein and surrounding tissues appear red, warm and swollen, and feel either tender or hard. Phlebitis may also be caused by mechanical or chemical irritation from the cannula or infusion fluid.
	Thrombophlebitis has the same signs and symptoms as uncomplicated phlebitis except that macro- or microscopic suppuration of the inflamed area develops. Pus may even drain from the infected entrance wound. Development of a subsequent high-grade bacteraemia is a decided possibility. This may necessitate surgical dissection of the inflamed vein/artery.
	Cellulitis is characterised by the development of oedema accompanied by warmth, tenderness and redness of the skin surrounding the entrance wound. Infusion fluid may possibly be a source of infection, especially when ingredients are added to existing solutions in patient care departments.
	Peripheral intravenous cannulas need to be changed every 48–72 hours, if possible, to avoid colonisation of the devices with pathogens. Central venous lines are to be evaluated and the entrance wounds cleaned every 48–72 hours. Daily observation and evaluation of the entrance wound is of extreme importance to identify the development of infection.
General signs and symptoms:	Phlebitis, purulent thrombophlebitis, cellulitis, drainage of pus from the puncture wound, pyrexia, pain or loss of sensation in the inflamed area is common in cannula-related infections.
Diagnosis:	Clinical signs and symptoms of purulent thrombophlebitis or cellulitis are an indication of infection. Cannula-related infections such as bacteraemia are difficult to diagnose in the absence of a clinical host reaction. Often microscopic analysis of the tip of the cannula or drainage from the entrance wound is the only method of confirming the presence of infection or identifying the causative micro-organism. Because colonisation of devices occurs quickly, a definite diagnosis of septicaemia is only made if the device culture is **confirmed** by two simultaneous blood cultures taken from different venous sites with similar growth.

Complications: Cellulitis, phlebitis/thrombophlebitis, extensive bacteraemia with resultant septicaemia, arterial or venous occlusion, loss of limbs and even death is possible due to cannula-related infections.

If contaminated infusate(s) or specially prepared solutions (e.g. parenteral hyperalimentation) are the cause of the infection, the first patient may be the index case of an outbreak of infection.

Strict aseptic technique must be used to commence infusions or to change sets/vaculiters.
The skin of the new site must be carefully disinfected with povidon iodine, an alcohol-based antiseptic, or 0,5% chlorhexidine gluconate in 70% alcohol. The disinfected skin should be touched as little as possible. All residual disinfectant must have evaporated before the device is passed through the skin or the occlusive dressing is sealed over the puncture area.

Opened intravenous devices and administering sets must be handled as little as possible to prevent contamination. To avoid contamination/soiling, the opened and unprotected end of the device should never be placed directly on the patient's bed. Intravenous administering sets must be changed every 48–72 hours, as micro-organism growth in the set may become a problem, unless a needleless infusion system with valved ports is used. These systems can be used for the duration specified by the manufacturer, usually a week.

Administering sets for parenteral hyperalimentation must be changed at least every 24 hours. After administering lipids, blood or blood products, the set has to be changed before any other type of fluid is transfused.

The rubber reservoirs of an administering set must never be 'pumped'. Small blood clots, crystalised trace elements and clumps of micro-organisms adhering to the end of the intravenous device will be forced into the patient's blood circulation and may form the basis of future thrombi.

Covering the entrance wound of the device with an occlusive, transparent dressing facilitates daily monitoring for signs of local infection and redness. The skin should be disinfected for 10mm beyond where the dressing will end, to prevent migration of skin organisms under the dressing.

Intravenous fluids and additives must be unclouded/clear before transfusion. Cloudy fluids may be a sign of contamination. All infusions such as self-produced ('home-made') aseptic parenteral hyperalimentation must be marked with the name and record number of the patient, the contents and expiry date. Refer also to the discussions on practice and procedures contained in chapters 6–8.

CONTROL/PREVENTATIVE MEASURES

Barrier measures		Protective clothing		Housekeeping	
Hand washing	✓	Gloves	✓	Cleaning	R
Hand disinfection	✓	Masks		Medical waste	R
Single room		Caps		Laundry	R
Private room + b/room		Eye protection			
Separate equipment	✓	Cotton gowns			
Limit visitors		Plastic aprons	✓		

Legal notification		Readily communicable in the healthcare setting	
On suspicion of infection		Yes	
On lab confirmation		No	✓

R = Routine   S = Special

UPPER RESPIRATORY TRACT INFECTIONS
e.g. sinusitis, parotitis, otitis media

Definition:

Hospital-acquired upper respiratory tract infections develop in the airways above and including the vocal cords after the patient has been hospitalised for a minimum of 48 hours or longer.

The most important hospital-acquired upper respiratory tract infections include:

Sinusitis: Inflammation of the paranasal sinuses due to infection caused by bacteria/viruses/fungi or allergic reactions.

Pharyngitis (sore throat): Inflammation of the throat, mostly due to viral or bacterial infections (e.g. Group A β-haemolytic streptococcus, staphylococcus or pneumococcus).

Acute otitis media: A bacterial or viral infection of the middle ear, usually as result of an upper respiratory tract infection.

Discussion:

Acute sinusitis may follow an acute viral respiratory infection, but is usually caused by pneumococci, staphylococci or streptococci. Chronic sinusitis may also be caused by irritation from chemical, mineral or vegetable sources such as gas fumes, perfume or cigarette smoke. Intubation with nasogastric or endotracheal tubes contributes to the risk of sinusitis, caused by contamination of the neighbouring maxillary sinus.

Acute pharyngitis is mainly caused by the drying out of the throat's mucosa, mechanical trauma (bronchoscopy/endotracheal intubation) or infection. Pharyngitis mainly causes discomfort which is seldom of great significance, unless more than one patient from the same patient-care area complains.

Acute otitis media is generally found amongst children aged 3 years or younger. Micro-organisms migrate from the infected nasopharynx (upper respiratory tract) to the middle ear via the mucosa of the Eustachian tube. Ear infection is a lesser known complication of endotracheal or nasogastric intubation.

General signs and symptoms:

Acute and chronic sinusitis has similar signs and symptoms:

Tenderness, pain and swelling in the area of the affected sinus(es); sometimes toothache; headache and malaise. The nasal mucosa is red and swollen, while the secretions may be offensive, viscous and coloured green or yellow. Fever and rigor may be due to the spread of the infection to other parts of the upper respiratory tract or the cranium.

Acute pharyngitis is characterised by a sore throat and painful swallowing. Swollen mucosa; hoarseness; fever; and swollen lymph glands in the neck and jaw are common. A hyperproduction of purulent mucus accompanies overt infection.

Acute otitis media is characterised by severe and continuous earache, loss of hearing, fever, diarrhoea, nausea and vomiting in children, red and swollen eardrums, purulent or bloodstained ear secretions, possible perforation of the tympanic membrane, accompanied by immediate relief from the pain that is characteristic of acute otitis media.

Diagnosis: Clinical signs and symptoms, the medical history of the patient, X-ray examination of sinuses as well as microbiological analysis of the secretions/sinus drainage to confirm the diagnosis and positively identify the causative organism(s). Taking throat swabs for laboratory analysis is a (largely) futile exercise unless the procedure is completed (and the specimen is handled) aseptically throughout. Throat swabs must be soaked in the secretion(s) and sent to the laboratory as quickly as possible to prevent drying out.

Complications: **Sinusitis:** Development of meningitis, otitis, tooth abscesses, hypertrophia of the mucosa and chronic maxillary sinusitis.

Pharyngitis: Usually no long-term complications.

Otitis media: Meningitis, permanent, partial or complete deafness, mastoiditis, facial paralysis, brain or epidural abscesses, subdural empyema as well as lateral sinus thrombosis are some of the more serious complications that occur when an ear infection is neglected or inappropriately treated.

CONTROL/PREVENTATIVE MEASURES					
Barrier measures		**Protective clothing**		**Housekeeping**	
Hand washing	✓	Gloves	✓	Cleaning	R
Hand disinfection	✓	Masks		Medical waste	R
Single room		Caps		Laundry	R
Private room + b/room		Eye protection			
Separate equipment		Cotton gowns			
Limit visitors		Plastic aprons	✓		

Legal notification		**Readily communicable in the healthcare setting**	
On suspicion of infection		Yes	
On lab confirmation		No	✓

R = Routine   S = Special

ENTERIC CONDITIONS (DIARRHOEA)

Definition: An increase in the nature and frequency of bowel movements that is perceived as abnormal by the afflicted person. The condition develops after a minimum of 48 hours following admission to hospital.

Discussion: Diarrhoea is mostly the symptom of an underlying condition such as food poisoning or an infection with bacteria/parasites/viruses. Changes in the diet, differences in osmolality of fluid diets, unprotected or excessive use of antimicrobials, oral medication, malabsorption of food, pathology of the intestines and increased peristalsis of the gastric tract may also cause diarrhoea. Food poisoning may be accompanied by diarrhoea caused by the toxins secreted by the infecting micro-organisms and the damaged tissue of the host. Diarrhoea is commonly spread by the unwashed hands of the infected person after a bowel movement. The spread of enteric conditions is common in communities with a lack of running water, overcrowding, poor sanitation and poor personal hygiene. Outbreaks of diarrhoea are generally found if food and water are contaminated with excreta.

When four or more persons contract food poisoning from the same source, the condition becomes a legally notifiable disease.

General signs and symptoms: A person normally passes stool between 2–3 times per day to 2–3 times per week. An increase/change in frequency, volume, consistency, odour or colour, as well as the presence of blood, pus, mucus or excessive fat in the stool, may indicate disease. Fever, electrolyte imbalance, prostration or vomiting may be found.

Diagnosis: Clinical evaluation is based on the aetiology, duration and severity of the diarrhoea, the medical history, clinical signs and symptoms as well as laboratory analysis to identify and prescribe treatment against the causative micro-organism(s).

Complications: Metabolic acidosis and electrolyte imbalance (mainly of sodium, potassium, magnesium, organic anions and chloride), loss of fluid and dehydration (which may be fatal in children), as well as vascular collapse, may be the result of continuous diarrhoea. Early rehydration and electrolyte replacement is necessary, especially in children (5 ml table salt, 5 ml bicarbonate of soda, and 20 ml sugar, dissolved in 1 litre of boiled, cooled water may be used as an oral rehydration solution).

CONTROL/PREVENTATIVE MEASURES

Barrier measures		Protective clothing		Housekeeping	
Hand washing	✓	Gloves	✓	Cleaning	R
Hand disinfection	✓	Masks		Medical waste	R
Single room (as necessary)	✓	Caps		Laundry	R
Private room + b/room (if applicable)	✓	Eye protection			
Separate equipment	✓	Cotton gowns			
Limit visitors	✓	Plastic aprons	✓		

Legal notification		Readily communicable in the healthcare setting	
On suspicion of infection		Yes in cases of poor hygienic conditions	✓
On lab confirmation		No	

R = Routine   S = Special

LOWER RESPIRATORY TRACT INFECTIONS e.g. *bronchitis, pneumonia*

Definition:

A hospital-acquired infection of the lower bronchial tract (below the larynx) that develops after a minimum of 48 hours following admission to hospital. The most significant of these infections include:

Pneumonia: A lung infection of primary or secondary origin (due to complication of another condition or invasive procedure such as endotracheal intubation). One or both lungs may be affected partially or totally.

Bronchitis: An acute or chronic condition caused by infecting micro-organisms, mechanical irritation (following an invasive procedure) or inhalation of an irritating gas/material.

Discussion:

Lower respiratory tract infections unfortunately are a reasonably common occurrence in hospitals. The elderly (65 years and older) and the very young (6 months and younger) are especially prone to this type of infection. Patients on mechanical ventilation, the bedridden, those who have undergone major trauma or extended anaesthesia/operations as well as immunosuppressed persons are at (high) risk of contracting hospital-acquired respiratory infections. Bacteria (especially staphylococcus and pneumococcus) and viruses normally found in the upper respiratory tract cause infections in the lower respiratory tract of susceptible patients. Drops, nasopharyngeal secretions as well as direct/oral contact with an afflicted carrier may transmit the causative pathogens from person- to-person or from the person to the environment. The infection usually remains contagious as long as viable organisms are present in the secretions.

General signs and symptoms:

Pneumonia: Fever, rigor, chills, sweating, a dry or productive cough, laborious breathing, increased tempo of respiration, pleural or substernal pain, respiratory discomfort or distress, consolidation of the lung tissues, headache, nausea and vomiting, confusion in the elderly or in children, prostration, myalgia, a sore throat, hoarseness, bloodstained sputum.

Aspiration pneumonia sometimes occurs during or just after birth, anaesthesia, during alcoholic intoxication, convulsions, extreme prostration (frailty) or during disturbances in consciousness due to vomiting or drowning.

Pneumocystis carinii pneumonia ('PCP') is strongly associated with immunosuppression in persons on mechanical ventilation, steroid therapy or those infected with the human immunodeficiency virus (HIV).

Bronchitis: An infection of more limited extent. A productive cough with bloodstained or purulent sputum develops within hours after exposure. Dyspnoea due to obstruction of the airways may occur. Similar symptoms to those of pneumonia are common, but develop to a lesser extent. Bronchopneumonia is diagnosed if the infection extends to the lungs.

Diagnosis:	Clinical signs and symptoms, the medical history, chest X-rays to detect consolidation of the lung tissues, microbiological laboratory analysis to confirm the diagnosis and to positively identify the causative micro-organism(s). **WARNING:** In very frail, elderly or paediatric patients, as well as the severely immunosuppressed, many of the traditionally acknowledged clinical signs and symptoms of pneumonia or bronchitis may be absent. An increased rate of respiration without pyrexia may be the only sign of the infection.
Complications:	**Pneumonia:** Bronchiolitis, meningitis, endocarditis, anoxia with brain damage (children), bacteraemia, a permanent degree of hypoxia, empyema, and death in extremely frail patients. **Bronchitis:** Complications usually occur in patients with underlying chronic respiratory disease. Chronic bronchitis may lead to emphysema, abnormal blood gas values or chronic airway disease.

CONTROL/PREVENTATIVE MEASURES						
Barrier measures		**Protective clothing**		**Housekeeping**		
Hand washing	✓	Gloves	✓	Cleaning		R
Hand disinfection	✓	Masks		Medical waste		R
Single room		Caps		Laundry		R
Private room + b/room		Eye protection				
Separate equipment		Cotton gowns				
Limit visitors		Plastic aprons	✓			

Legal notification		**Readily communicable in the healthcare setting**	
On suspicion of infection		Yes	
On lab confirmation		No	✓

R = Routine   S = Special

URINARY TRACT INFECTIONS

Definition: The presence of abnormal counts of pathogenic micro-organisms in the urine, causing a clinical/microscopic perceptible host reaction that develops a minimum of 48 hours or longer after admission to the hospital.

Discussion: Urinary tract infection is the most common type of hospital-acquired infection. This includes nephritis, cystitis and urethritis. Usually these are acute infections although chronic urinary tract infection may flare up if the susceptible patient is exposed to 'new' micro-organisms. Females are 10 times more prone to urinary tract infections than males. Most urinary tract infections are bacterial in nature. Gram-negative infections are the most difficult to eradicate. The incidence of fungal and viral infections is relatively low, except in immunosuppressed patients. Caregivers' hands are regularly contaminated with urine when continuous urine drainage bags or collection containers are emptied. Impeccable hand hygiene and the use of gloves is essential for the continued health of the worker. Clean, dry equipment for the mass collection/drainage of urine bags is necessary to contain the spread of (cross-) infection amongst patients or staff members.

General signs and symptoms: A burning sensation or painful micturition, frequency (with small volumes of urine), suprapubic discomfort with/without pelvic or lower-back pain, nocturia, pyuria, haematuria with/without offensive urine, pyrexia.

Diagnosis: Microbiological analysis is necessary to confirm the diagnosis, positively identify the causative micro-organism(s) and indicate treatment. A count of at least 100 000 or more colony-forming units of micro-organisms per ml of urine (cfu/ml) is indicative of urinary tract infection **if** a specimen was obtained:

- from the distal end of the catheter, or
- after disinfection, with a sterile needle and syringe from the sample site of the catheter's drainage tube, or
- aseptically as a midstream ('clean catch') specimen.

The presence of large numbers of three or more types of bacteria in a specimen may indicate contamination or the incorrect storage of the collected urine. In the case of a patient with long-term continuous catheterisation, a high micro-organism unit count may be seen as normal. Urine specimens with less than 100 000 cfu/ml may be due to colonisation rather than overt infection, depending on the individual patient.

Complications: Chronic/recurring urinary tract infection due to unsuitable, insufficient or uncompleted antibiotic treatment; urethral- or bladder neck strictures; bladder or renal stones; hydronephrosis due to obstruction of the ureters and/or bladder in extreme cases; haemorrhagic cystitis accompanied by anaemia, chronic bacteriuria, chronic renal failure, acute bacterial prostatitis and/or epididymitis in male patients, ulcerating urethritis.

CONTROL/PREVENTATIVE MEASURES					
Barrier measures		**Protective clothing**		**Housekeeping**	
Hand washing	✓	Gloves	✓	Cleaning	R
Hand disinfection	✓	Masks		Medical waste	R
Single room		Caps		Laundry	R
Private room + b/room		Eye protection			
Separate equipment	✓	Cotton gowns			
Limit visitors		Plastic aprons	✓		

Legal notification		**Readily communicable in the healthcare setting**	
On suspicion of infection		Yes	
On lab confirmation		No	✓

R = Routine   S = Special

A REVIEW OF WOUND INFECTIONS AND WOUND CARE

Definition: Infection usually presents as a purulent discharge in an open wound or as an enclosed cavity filled with pus. The pus contains viable pathogens/ potential pathogens, causing a **clinically perceptible host reaction**. Hospital-acquired wound infections develop 48 hours or longer after surgery or admission to hospital.

Discussion: Wound infection is the second most common type of infection in patient-care areas. Burns carry the highest risk of morbidity and mortality of all the wounds, especially in children or patients with a burnt body surface of 30% or more.

The protection against infection afforded by the patient's skin is destroyed by trauma, surgical incision, contamination/soiling, a penetrating accident or inoculation with micro-organisms (e.g. needle pricks). This is followed by further invasion and multiplication of the micro-organisms/pathogens in the host's tissues. When this process takes place, a clinically perceptible host reaction follows. Often the source of infection is the patient's own skin or enteric flora (an endogenous infection), transmitted by himself or a caregiver to a susceptible infection site. Exogenous infection is transmitted from an external source such as contaminated instruments, medication, linen or another person's hands. Staphylococcus, Gram-negative bacilli (e.g. *E. coli*), streptococcus, klebsiella, clostridium and pseudomonas are some of the most common causes of wound infection.

Tracing the cause(s) of hospital-acquired wound infections is time consuming. It includes:

- identifying what caused the wound
- the duration of operations/surgery
- what pre-operative preparation, if any, was given
- location of the wound (e.g. the gastric tract)
- the use of antibiotics or antiseptics before, during or after surgery
- the vascular response of the patient
- foreign objects placed in the wound, such as sutures or drains
- the volume and type of drainage from the wound
- wound care procedures/techniques
- what type of dressing was used on the wound
- who was present and what they did.

Patients and staff members continuously shed microscopically small flakes of skin and hair. These flakes may fall into open wounds during surgery or wound care procedures, causing contamination and (cross-) infection as each flake may carry as many as 100 or more individual staphylococci. Staff members must therefore be aware of the risk and take all possible precautions (including wearing caps and face masks during wound care procedures to protect the susceptible patient).

General signs and symptoms:	**Deep wounds:** Localised erythema, vesicles/pustules, pyrexia (localised or systemic), tenderness, swelling, pain/discomfort, ruptured suturing or incomplete wound healing, bacteraemia or a suppurating discharge from the wound. For various reasons, signs of localised inflammation may not be noticed immediately, i.e. they may be hidden by occlusive dressings or rashes from skin allergies. **Superficial wounds:** Similar manifestations as those of deeper wounds, but they may be less extensive and easier to see and treat.
Diagnosis:	Clinical identification is based on the wound aetiology, the patient's medical history, the duration and degree of infection as well as microbiological laboratory analysis.
Complications:	Severe scarring, bacteraemia/septicaemia, development of drug resistant micro-organisms (not sensitive to the usually prescribed antibiotics), poor wound healing, abscess development, necrosis, extended hospitalisation, cross-infection, debilitation, increased morbidity and mortality.

CONTROL/PREVENTATIVE MEASURES					
Barrier measures		**Protective clothing**		**Housekeeping**	
Hand washing	✓	Gloves	✓	Cleaning	R
Hand disinfection	✓	Masks (open wounds)	✓	Medical waste	R
Single room (open wounds)	✓	Caps (open wounds)	✓	Laundry	R
Private room + b/room		Eye protection			
Separate equipment	✓	Cotton gowns			
Limit visitors		Plastic aprons (open wounds)	✓		

Legal notification		Readily communicable in the healthcare setting	
On suspicion of infection		Yes	
On lab confirmation		No	✓

R = Routine   S = Special

Wound care procedures

The following paragraphs offer a short review of the highlights and problems in applying infection prevention and control measures in wound care procedures.

Wound dressings

The choice of appropriate wound dressings is becoming more difficult due to the glut of good-quality, sterile, single-use products available today. The problem is one of choice: many look similar but work differently, or are composite dressings with a combination of functions depending on the nature of the wound.

Classification

- **Semi-permeable adhesive dressings** are 'breathing' transparent films, coated with adhesive and made from polyurethane, for use on minor burns, lacerations, stage 1 pressure sores, post–operative wounds, and entrance sites of peripheral and central venous lines. Some examples: OpSite® (for wounds), OpSite IV 3000® (for intravascular catheter entrance sites), Tegaderm® or Bioclusive®.

- **Hydrocolloid wafers** and pastes are dressings with a hydrophilic hydrocolloid base containing different ingredients in an adhesive hydrophobic polymer matrix. The outer layer of these dressings is either a waterproof film or a combination of waterproof polyurethane foams and films that prevent strike-through. These dressings are used on partial-thickness wounds, clean stage 3 and 4 pressure sores, necrotic and sloughy wounds, and mild to moderately exuding wounds. Some examples: Comfeel®, Granuflex®, Replicare®, Tegasorb®, Hydrocol®.

- **Hydrogels** consist of gel-forming polymer, water and propylene glycol. These dressings are supplied in tubes, foil packets, spray bottles, impregnated gauze pads or as sheets on a thin fibre mesh, for use on partial- and full-thickness wounds (such as stage 2–4 pressures sores), necrotic and sloughy wounds, burns, wounds with hollows (dead spaces), for debridement and/or softening of eschar. Some examples: IntraSite Gel®, IntraSite Conformable®, Granugel®, Nu-Gel®.

- **Absorption or filler dressings** are highly absorbent dressings, some of which are made of:
  - a non-woven composite of calcium alginate fibres (a cellulose-like polysaccaride), e.g. Kaltostat®
  - hydrofibre, e.g. Aquacel® 3M foam.

These dressings are intended for use on moderate to extensively exuding wounds, e.g. donor sites, leg ulcers, pressure sores, fungating wounds, wounds with combined necrosis, high exudation and/or infection, and wounds that require packing and absorption.

- **Semi-permeable polyurethane foam dressings** have a hydrophilic action that provides a low-adherent wound contact layer, while others have a hydrophobic moisture-vapour permeable backing that prevents strike-through. The edges of the dressing show when the dressing is saturated. These dressings are intended for use on partial- to full-thickness wounds with minimal to moderate exudates, or as secondary dressings for wounds requiring additional absorption and around drainage tubes. Some examples: Allevyn®/Allevyn Adhesive®/Allevyn Cavity®, Tielle®, Lyofoam®.

- **Odour-absorbing dressings** are low-adherent dressings containing either activated charcoal cloth or activated carbon to reduce wound odour. They are intended for use on malodorous wounds, e.g. fungating carcinomas, leg ulcers, or infected wounds with low to moderate exudates. Some examples include Actisorb Plus® and Lyofoam C®.

- **Impregnated gauze dressings** are open impregnated mesh, cotton, rayon, viscose or gauze dressings containing either soft paraffin, antiseptic or antibacterial agents, intended for use on superficial wounds (abrasions, lacerations, leg ulcers), wounds in the later stages of healing, and/or lightly exuding wounds, and to treat and/or counter infection. Some examples include Jelonet®, Bactigras®, Grassolind®, Sofratulle®.

- **Unmedicated gauze dressings** (e.g. plain gauze or cellulose dressings) are used for lightly to moderately exuding wounds; wounds with tunnelling, sinus tracts or dead spaces requiring packing; and exuding wounds containing necrosis.

- **Iodine-containing dressings** such as:
  - knitted viscose dressings impregnated with 10% povidone-iodine in a water-soluble polyethylene glycol base, e.g. Inadine®
  - Cadexomer iodine (CI) dressings consisting of a starch lattice of spherical microbeads impregnated with iodine at a concentration of 0.9% (v/v), e.g. Iodosorb®.

- **Silver-containing dressings** are antimicrobial dressings. They are intended for use on infected wounds and should be used as primary dressings. Examples include Acticoat®.
- **Home-made dressings**, including:
  - clean, washed and ironed cotton or linen squares or unsterile gauze placed on wounds after being baked in a dry oven for 60 minutes at 160°C, or ironed repeatedly at a high temperature and placed on the wound while still warm
  - cotton wool wrapped in clean, washed and ironed cotton or linen (must not come into contact with the wound bed)
  - clean sanitary towels (never inserted into a wound, but positioned on top for maximum absorption).

It must be emphasised that the use of any commercial dressing should always be in accordance with the specific manufacturer's instructions, to ensure safe and optimal results. Furthermore, the choice of dressing should always be determined by the nature of a wound, after a thorough and holistic assessment of the patient and the wound.

Protective clothing

Using protective clothing correctly has a mutual shielding effect for both the patient and the staff member, e.g. sterile gloves are used to protect the patient from micro-organisms while unsterile gloves are used to protect the wearer from contamination. Masks protect the wearer from splashes to the face and airways, as well as inspiration of drops and contaminated aerosols exhaled by the patient. Caps keep the caregiver's hair out of the wound, but also protect the wearer from drops from the patient, that land on the hair and head, dry out and then later splinter off, only to land on sterile work areas and the scrubbed hands of the person who bends down to work. Using protective clothing proactively when there is an assessed risk of contamination protects the staff and patient from being contaminated during a procedure. Patients with extensive cancer, those on long-term steroid therapy, or with full-blown AIDS are more susceptible to infection carried by the caregiver due to the depression of their own immunity, and must be protected. There are a few alternatives that can be used in place of traditional protective clothing when in a home-based care setting (refer to chapter 10 – 'Infection control in home-based care settings').

Barrier nursing is combined with the use of protective clothing to protect the patient, staff member and the environment. This simple flow-chart will help the caregiver to decide which infection prevention and control measures are appropriate to combat the assessed level of infection risk.

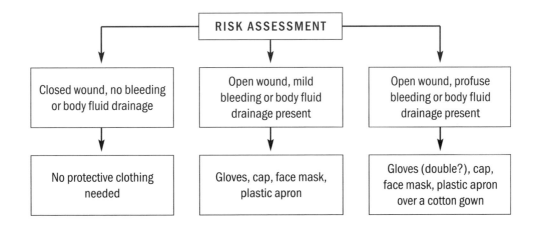

Technique

The technique of wound care will depend on the needs of the patient, the assessment of the wound, the demands of asepsis, the procedures and policies of the employing authority, the available supplies and services such as steam sterilisation, the environment and situation in which the work is to be performed, as well as the skill of the caregiver. If sterile supplies, equipment and instruments are available they should be used, but in situations where there are not even unsterile gloves available, procedures should be changed from working with washed, gloved hands to using non-touch techniques with washed hands and disinfected instruments such as forceps. Commercial disinfectants or sterilants such as the aldehydes or peracetic acid can be used in closed containers in the boot of a car to sterilise washed instruments (or at least disinfect them to a high-level) while travelling between patients during home-based care. Rinsing them with chlorinated drinking water (municipal tap water) before the next use is a good compromise to using a new set of sterile instruments for each patient.

The table below shows some alternatives which may be used in wound care when in a home-based care setting.

Item	Alternative 1	Alternative 2
Gloves, latex or vinyl	Kitchen gloves, reusable, washable	Intact plastic bags over the hands
Plastic aprons	Plastic waste bags, cut open	Plastic rain coat or rubberised overalls
Masks	Head or neck kerchief knotted over airways	Recycled cotton or linen offcuts
Caps	Head or neck kerchief knotted over hair	Shower cap
Linen savers	Cut-open plastic waste bags under a sheet	Layers of old newspaper under a sheet
Sterile gloves	Sterile instruments (non-touch technique)	Washed and disinfected instruments (non- touch technique)
Antiseptic solution for wound irrigation	5 ml table salt dissolved in 750 ml of boiled, cooled water	1 part vinegar in 18 parts boiled, cooled water
	5 ml Epson salts dissolved in 750 ml of boiled, cooled water	Rehydration fluid: 5 ml table salt, 5 ml bicarbonate of soda, and 20 ml sugar, dissolved in 1litre of boiled, cooled water
Powdered gloves	Baby talc in kitchen gloves	Corn starch
Commercial disinfectant/sterilant for instruments	Pasteurisation (Chapter 5)	Disinfection (Chapter 5)

Section Two
Infection control practice

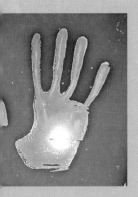

In this section a selection of infection control practices that form the basis of safe patient care and personnel safety are discussed in detail. These measures are universally applicable. The most important points are illustrated as these usually form the weak link in the infection control chain. Healthcare workers should consult the section on informed consent on page 221 before undertaking any procedure.

The objectives of this section are to:
- Ensure that all staff apply standard/set infection prevention and control measures when caring for patients with infections.
- Ensure that all staff are protected from occupationally acquired infections when caring for patients with infections.
- Facilitate auditing of patient records and care standards.
- Facilitate costing structures and cost-effective nursing care.
- Facilitate auditing of accounts.

The following outcomes are expected if the policies and procedures discussed in this section are applied:
- Trained staff care for patients who are immunosuppressed or patients with suspected or confirmed infection.
- Standard/set measures are applied by all nursing and supporting staff over a 24-hour period when caring for immuno-suppressed patients or patients with suspected or confirmed infection.
- Cost-effective care of a high standard is ensured.
- Attention is paid to patient care, occupational health, and staff safety as well as environmental measures.
- Staff are protected during caregiving by applying scientifically proven infection prevention and control measures.

Scope of practice
- Policies and procedures are applicable to all healthcare personnel in patient-care units.
- Appropriate isolation equipment and supplies are freely available.
- An infection control service is resident in the hospital and available for consultation about appropriate isolation measures OR written guidelines are available to all staff for application of policies.
- Visitors fall under the direct supervision of the patient-care unit staff.

4 | Housekeeping

Hospital and environmental hygiene

Though the environment plays a limited role in the transmission of infection, a dirty patient-care area actively maintains and promotes infection. The purpose of cleaning is to physically and effectively remove micro-organisms from surfaces and fomites that may be involved in the transmission of infection from patient to patient or patient to personnel/environment. In areas where highly susceptible patients such as infants, children or immunosuppressed patients are cared for, the environment does become a factor to take into account. Due to the effect of gravity and activity, the floor is the most soiled environment in any healthcare facility. Recuperating toddlers and bigger children play on the floor, often before (all) the symptoms of infection have cleared up and before the children are pathogen-free. It is therefore essential that particular care be taken in vulnerable areas.

Definition. Cleaning is the physical removal of soiling/contamination such as organic matter from surfaces, leaving them safe for use. Only the very best methods with the best equipment available are good enough for cleaning hospitals and healthcare facilities.

Cleaning is the first step in lowering the biological environmental load. Soap and warm water combined with 'elbow grease' is the most effective, simplest and cheapest method of removing up to 80% of transient environmental micro-organisms. Sterilisation and disinfection (e.g. pasteurisation) are only effective after surfaces or objects have been

thoroughly cleaned. Most patient-care areas can be adequately cleaned using detergent and warm water, but not the following high-risk patient-care areas:

- procedure/dressing rooms
- neonatal care units
- patient isolation rooms
- operating theatres
- theatre suites
- intensive care units
- maternity and paediatric wards
- laboratories
- casualty departments
- oncology specialist units
- central sterilisation departments.

Prescribing special cleaning methods for high-risk areas (but not for others) implies that a certain level of dirt is acceptable in the other areas. High-risk areas where immuno-suppressed patients are present may require additional disinfection; the reason for this additional protection is the need to remove a slightly higher percentage of live micro-organisms from the environment.

General cleaning methods

Washing

- One part liquid detergent is added to 200–500 parts warm water. A thin layer of foam should form on the water's surface. In areas where the water is hard, more detergent might be needed. Too much detergent in the water makes surfaces sticky, necessitating recleaning.
- Detergents loosen adhered transient

micro-organisms from surfaces. Friction in turn removes up to 80% of these loosened micro-organisms, transferring them to washing cloths or cleaning equipment.

- No additives (such as scourers, disinfectants or floor polish) must be mixed with the detergent and water, as this deactivates the active cleaning ingredients in the detergent.
- Clean cloths must be issued daily as soiled cleaning equipment only spreads contamination.
- Deodorising is needed less often if drains, sluice rooms and used equipment are kept clean and as dry as possible.

Damp dusting

- Dry dusting is ineffectual and only displaces dust. Dusting is always done with a **damp** cloth, kept especially for dusting.
- One part liquid detergent is added to 1000 parts warm water to break the surface tension of the water, allowing dust particles to cling to natural or synthetic dusting cloths. Friction causes the build-up of an electrical charge on the surfaces being dusted. Consequent-ly, dust is drawn back to the charged object.
- Dust contains large numbers of micro-organisms such as bacilli and staphylococci as well as the dried nuclei of bacteria such as *Mycobacterium tuberculosis*. Inhaling contaminated dust may be more infectious than contact with sputum containing this bacillus as a larger infecting dose can be transmitted in this manner.
- Dust readily clings to and contaminates woolly and woven surfaces (carpets, curtains, bedding, and the jerseys and clothes of health care workers).
- Dusting equipment must be clean.
- Only clean surfaces can be dusted with any success.
- Feather dusters are absolutely banned from healthcare facilities as they only displace dust.

Sweeping

- Sweeping is completed using long strokes of a clean cotton or synthetic mop, pushed along the floor without being picked up or shaken. This keeps the dust at floor level.
- Ordinary brooms should be banished from hospitals as the individual bristles only displace dust and disturb the air, causing flurries that deposit the dust elsewhere.
- Mops should have detachable heads for machine-washing at 65°C–75°C (145°F–170°F) (pasteurisation) before drying. Alternatively the heads can be covered with disposable cloths and dampened with the dusting solution to improve dust control.
- Sweeping smooth floors with a synthetic mop builds up an electric charge that attracts dust. Damp-sweeping floors improves dust containment.
- Loose litter must be collected and not just pushed along the floor.
- Only relatively clean floors can be swept. Soiled floors require washing.
- External floors and paving should be washed with a hose and water under pressure and not swept.
- Pedestrian areas that are being cleaned must be clearly indicated, especially wet and slippery floors.

Vacuuming

- Vacuum cleaners must be equipped with proper filters to ensure that micro-organisms, which are drawn into the machine, are contained and not just blown out through the exhaust vents again.
- The dust reservoir must be cleaned and washed out daily.
- Salmonella may survive for months in a dusty environment and can be disseminated through poor housekeeping.
- Over-filling the machine or paper collection bag should be avoided as this will only spread and not collect the dust. Filled paper

bags must be discarded and not reused.

- Unsoiled curtains may be vacuumed, reducing the need for laundering.

Disinfection

- Disinfecting equipment such as mops and dusting cloths is ineffectual because cotton and synthetic materials deactivate disinfectants. It therefore only leads to a false sense of security about the hygiene of the cleaning equipment.
- Environmental disinfection may be just as problematic because dust and organic matter also deactivate disinfectants. If a surface has been soiled/contaminated with organic matter (such as human body fluid or blood), the following two-step disinfection procedure must be initiated:
  1. Wash the area using soap and water, then rinse and dry, preferably with disposable paper towels.
  2. Apply disinfectant with a clean cloth and leave to air-dry spontaneously.
- Disinfectants are not deodorisers and should not be used as such. Micro-organisms loose their sensitivity to disinfectants if they are often exposed to the chemicals.
- Dusting with a disinfectant is ineffectual and costly as the small volumes evaporate quickly without enough time for disinfection. Even a small amount of dust and organic matter causes deactivation of disinfectants.
- Usually floors only require washing with soap and warm water. Washed and disinfected floors will re colonise with the original number of micro-organisms. No permanent reduction in biological levels can be achieved on floors and micro-organisms will recolonise on disinfected floors within an hour. The higher the level of activity and the number of contaminating feet/wheels, the quicker the original levels of contamination will be regained.

General hints for cleaning

- Cleaning equipment in the hands of careless workers makes cleaning a meaningless task.
- Poor cleaning procedures can lead to self-infection and cross-infection.
- Education in the principles of cleaning and hygiene, regular in-service training and constant supervision are required to make cleaning meaningful.
- Written policies and instructions act as guidelines for new staff members who are still uncertain about procedures.
- Regular hand-washing is essential for cleaning staff. Working with soap does not guarantee clean hands as soap itself is easily contaminated. Micro-organisms such as pseudomonas and Gram-negative bacilli grow actively in soiled soap.
- Protective clothing: cleaning staff should make use of protective clothing such as commercial gloves, waterproof aprons and shoes when working in potentially contaminated patient-care areas.
- Dust-free walls usually carry few micro-organisms. Obvious soiling and contamination with human body fluid or blood must be washed off walls as soon as possible. Regular washing and especially disinfection leads to corrosion and cracking of paint or wall coverings, offering shelter to micro-organisms.
- Ceilings carry a small infection risk and need cleaning only when soiled. An annual cleaning to remove dust on loose panelled ceilings may be necessary.
- Electricity attracts dust, so electric lights, ceiling fittings and wall-mounted electric equipment should be dusted as frequently as needed. Obvious soiling should be washed off the items after the electric current has been disconnected.
- Toilets: the outside and the inside (above the water level) of flush toilets should be

washed at least daily (and as necessary). The cleaners must wear gloves and use soap and water. The swirling action of flushing water removes most of the transient micro-organisms inside the toilet bowl. Contamination with organic matter, blood or body fluid on the outside, requires two-step disinfection (as detailed in the section on Disinfection on page 142) with an appropriate disinfectant.

- Toilet brushes often contain organic matter that cannot be rinsed from the bristles. Another brush is then needed to brush out the contents, risking contamination to the worker and environment. The contaminated water running from the brush usually collects in its container or stand, becoming a source of infection. The general use of toilet brushes in healthcare facilities must be considered in the light of the infection risk they pose.

- Sinks, sluices, washbasins and showers should be cleaned at least daily (and as necessary) with an all purpose cleaner, warm water and a soft brush. Scouring with an abrasive cleaner will leave microscopic scratches in enamel or stainless steel that will collect dirt and offer shelter to micro-organisms.

- Flushing a handful of washing-soda crystals and running hot water down drains once a week dissolves grease and cleans inside pipes where ordinary washing is impossible.

- Brushing overflows and grids with a small bottlebrush and a washing-soda solution will prevent scum buildup.

- Adding 20–50 ml of a 3% acetic acid solution to drainage pipes overnight will combat pseudomonas in theatres, burns and intensive care units.

- Bathtubs pose a unique infection risk. Disinfecting cleaned bathtubs after every use promotes patient protection. This is recommended, especially in maternity wards which have no amenities for Sitz bathing or wards where hydrotherapy is part of wound care.

- Clean water is required for cleaning. Used, dirty water does not clean, and will further contaminate the environment if used.

- Flowers and fish bowls: stagnant water from flower vases and aquariums may become a source of infection with Gram-negative micro-organisms and should be changed regularly. Topping up is unacceptable.

- Critical patient-care equipment is the domain of the nursing staff and should be cleaned by them. This includes incubators, mechanical respirators and ventilators, humidifiers as well as ordinary items such as shaving equipment, stethoscopes and digital thermometers. Again, the use of soap and water is indicated to remove organic matter, followed by either disinfection or a sterilisation method in high-risk patient care areas. Ordinary, non-disposable razors require disinfection and new blades for usage between patients. The use of disposable razors is strongly recommended.

- Mattresses and pillows with torn slipcovers are a source of infection from micro-organisms such as acinetobacter and other Gram-negatives. Waterproof covers should be acquired and the surfaces washed with soap and warm water, then wiped down after every patient discharge. Terminal disinfection may be required if the previous patient suffered from a contaminating or infectious condition.

- Liquid-soap bottles should be washed with a brush and warm water every second day, rinsed with hot water, drained and filled with enough soap for two days. Topping up is unacceptable as micro-organisms readily grow in contaminated soap. The micro-organisms are transferred to healthcare workers every time someone washes their hands and are then transmitted to patients.

- Urinals and bedpans should be rinsed with running cold water, washed with a brush and soap and water at least daily (and as necessary). After use, the inside of the emptied container should be rinsed with running cold water and the unsoiled exterior disinfected with an appropriate disinfectant from a spray bottle. Hypochlorite is active against many micro-organisms but is easily deactivated by organic matter. If a urinal or bedpan is emptied and only rinsed, invisible traces of organic matter, perspiration and scraps of human skin from the previous patient will still contaminate the external surface.
- Wet or damp equipment must be washed and dried before reuse. The level of success in cleaning partly depends on the hygienic condition of the equipment. In turn this depends on its treatment after previous use.
- Disposable cleaning equipment might be safer but adds to the volume of hospital waste. Reusable equipment must be handled with care to avoid contamination of the environment and the spread of infection.
- Mechanised equipment such as scrubbing machines, vacuum cleaners and floor polishers should be well maintained and repaired as soon as they break down. Broken equipment may damage floor coverings and surfaces, allowing potential pathogens to shelter and multiply in cracks and rough areas.
- Plastic equipment such as buckets, brushes, sponges and squeegees must be washed and dried, as micro-organisms readily adhere to synthetic materials, forming an invisible biofilm that may harbour pathogens. Hollow equipment, such as the cleaning reservoirs, pipes and tanks of scrubbing machines, should be drained, washed, rinsed and, if possible, inverted to allow drainage of fluids.

- Colour-coding plastic refuse bags to indicate high risk or normal household contents helps illiterate or inexperienced cleaning staff to dispose of potentially hazardous waste with care.
- Acquiring suitable cleaning agents is essential for hospital hygiene, especially where children or immunosuppressed patients are accommodated. Cleaning agents can be very costly. Expert advice is needed before purchasing a range of chemical agents, to ensure mutual compatibility and cleaning efficiency.
- Pest control (ants, rodents, flies, pigeons, cockroaches, and even stray dogs and cats) has to be combined with cleaning procedures, as the two are mutually dependent in hospital hygiene.

Hospital and environmental hygiene are extremely important aspects of infection control, and should be placed high on the list of priorities when formulating procedures. Cleaning staff must be properly trained and supervised in order to perform these essential tasks correctly. Your facility's administration staff must be made aware of correct infection control procedures.

Food handling

Outbreaks of food-borne infection in patient, care institutions usually affect many patients, staff members and visitors. Due to such factors as the use of antibiotics (which decreases the numbers of normal enteral flora in patients) gastric surgery, the use of antacids, extremes of age, malignancy or immunosuppression, hospitalised patients are at increased risk of acquiring food-borne infection. Small inocula of enteric pathogens that might be innocuous in most healthy individuals can cause disease and even death in highly susceptible patients.

You should note the following facts:

- Salmonella species are the most common cause of food poisoning (80%).
- The infective dose a healthy person must ingest to develop an enteric disease is about 10 000 micro-organisms.
- Bacillus species are found everywhere, but especially in cereals and dried food such as rice and spices.
- Bacillus produces a heat-resistant toxin that survives heating to 121°C for 90 minutes.
- If prepared contaminated food is stored at room temperature, the bacteria starts producing toxins.
- Clostridium is commonly found if leftover food is reheated but not boiled again.
- 50–70% of staphylococci produce enterotoxin, which induces vomiting and diarrhoea hours after ingesting sufficient numbers of the micro-organism.
- Food is usually prepared elsewhere, then transported and served in the patient-care areas.
- Three food preparation methods are generally used:
  1. Food is freshly cooked and kept above 60–63°C until served.
  2. Cook-freeze, where cooked food is cooled to -5°C within 90 minutes and stored at -18°C until reheated and served.
  3. Cook-chill, where cooked food is cooled and stored at 0–3°C for up to 5 or more days before reheating and serving. Most efficient food storage refrigerators should function at 4–10°C.
- Poor personal hygiene or faulty patient-care procedures may cause secondary transmission of enteric pathogens when healthcare workers or patients become infected and unknowingly expose other patients or staff members to infection.

For food-borne infections to develop into outbreaks, the prepared food must become infected with pathogens or their toxins.

Some prerequisites for the development of food-borne infections include the mismanagement of raw or prepared food, allowing contamination and multiplication of micro-organisms to take place before ingestion by susceptible patients. Prevention of outbreaks of food-borne disease is the only successful infection control measure. Institutions must take into account the problems of:

- handling large amounts of raw food
- accommodating and preparing different diets
- preparing and storing food before serving
- serving large quantities of food throughout the day
- planning meals for immunosuppressed or susceptible patients
- contamination of food by catering staff due to personal disease, such as enteric infection, or through lack of knowledge and foresight.

General hints for food management

Evaluating the quality of raw/unprepared food

- All meat must be inspected, even if bought from a certified source. Contamination of raw red meat is uncommon (<01%) but offal (kidneys, liver and heart) and products made from mixtures of meat from several carcasses (mince and sausages) are more likely to be contaminated.
- Milk is potentially extremely dangerous and must be obtained already pasteurised from a certified source. Bovine tuberculosis (*Mycobacterium bovis*) and brucellosis (*Brucella abortus*) may be transmitted to susceptible patients by raw milk.
- Soft cheese manufactured from unpasteurised milk may potentially infect the foetuses of pregnant women or immunosuppressed patients with listeria, causing meningitis and septicaemia.
- Only clean, unbroken eggs should be

purchased. Soiled eggs may be contaminated with salmonella and campylobacter, which penetrate the egg through cracks in the shell and the protecting cuticle.

- Fresh chicken should be purchased from a dependable source. More than half of all fresh carcasses are contaminated with salmonella and campylobacter from the gut of the animals. No other raw foodstuffs may be prepared on the unwashed/undisinfected surfaces on which the raw chicken has been handled.
- Frozen chicken is usually less contaminated than the fresh product. Those micro-organisms that are present will multiply when the carcass is slowly defrosted at room temperature (2–4 hours). Rapid microwave defrosting or overnight defrosting at 4–10°C (40–50°F) in a refrigerator is preferable. Cooking at 70°C for at least 5 minutes kills salmonella and campylobacter. Care should be taken that the whole chicken cooks through to the bone.

Efficient handling of unprepared food

- There is a greater risk of transmitting infection through mismanagement of food, than through infection from a sick staff member.
- Raw and cooked meat must be stored separately to prevent contamination of prepared dishes.
- The protection of supplies of raw or unprepared foodstuffs from environmental soiling or contact with unauthorised persons/pests is essential.
- Uncooked fruit, greens and vegetables used for salads should be washed and rinsed well before drying. Fruit that can be peeled (such as oranges and bananas) is safer to use than unpeeled fruit, especially for immunosuppressed patients. Uncooked salads and fruit such as grapes, or food such as dried biltong and processed cheese may cause fatal infections in highly immuno-

suppressed patients such as terminally ill AIDS patients.

Adequate cooking and refrigeration of prepared food

- Adequate cooking destroys most causative micro-organisms and some of the more heat-sensitive toxins.
- Pork should be cooked at 55°C (130°F) until no pink meat is visible near the bone. All pork products must be well cooked, especially if they are to be refrigerated for a few days and served cold. *Yersinia entercolitis*, which causes diarrhoea in humans and grows at 2°C (36°F), can multiply in refrigerated pork from a few bacteria to millions within 10 days.
- Cold and hot foods must be prepared in separate work areas to prevent contamination or cross-infection of the prepared dishes.
- Food that is eaten raw such as uncooked salads must be stored separately from unprepared food and cooked dishes, to avoid the possibility of accidental contamination.
- Cold foods should be stored at ±7°C (45°F) or lower temperatures to prevent the development of staphylococcal enterotoxin. Cooked foods should reach at least 74°C (165°F) throughout and be kept at 60°C (140°F) or higher.
- All food must be kept covered between preparation and serving.
- Food such as tuna salads, ham, chicken, eggs, home-made salad dressings and milk products that readily support bacterial growth should not be prepared more than three hours before serving and should never be held over from one meal to another.
- Prompt refrigeration of prepared food is essential.
- Unrefrigerated milk contaminated with *Bacillus cereus* is a major cause of food poisoning in hospitals as this micro-organism survives pasteurisation and refrigeration. Spoilt milk must be discarded without delay.

- Cooking eggs is the only protection against salmonella and campylobacter as they are harboured in the pores of eggshells. Raw eggs should not be used in patients' diets.
- Ice should be treated like any other food. It should never be scooped by hand directly from an ice machine.
- Food should not be kept on the ice inside an ice-making machine.
- No movement should be allowed between the different food preparation areas (e.g. where vegetable and meat preparation is done or freezing/chilling takes place) as cross-contamination between clean and contaminated work areas can readily occur.

Good personal hygiene

- All food handlers must be educated to achieve high standards of personal and environmental hygiene (hand-washing, the need for environmental cleanliness and the sanitary disposal of all waste from food preparation areas). The standards should be enforced by constant supervision.
- Most food-borne infections are due to contamination with salmonella (from hands) or staphylococci (from hands, unwashed skin, mouths or noses).
- Smoking and eating should be prohibited in food preparation areas.
- Pre-employment medical examination of food handlers is required, followed by periodic routine examinations.
- Staff with respiratory and especially enteral ailments must be excluded from direct food handling during illness (and for at least one week after a bout of diarrhoea). Enteric illness at home must be reported to the food manager or supervisor.
- Food handlers can be the carriers of micro-organisms without becoming ill themselves, e.g. streptococci may be sheltered in an asymptomatic carrier's nasopharynx.
- Open skin lesions should be covered with impermeable wound dressings, especially on the hands.
- The unpleasant habit of licking one's fingers to pick up food wrapping paper must be actively discouraged.
- Hands should be disinfected with a suitable hand rub or washed:
  - before food preparation, especially if no further cooking is required
  - after handling raw food
  - after handling a patient's leftover food or food waste
  - after visiting the cloakroom
  - every time the person coughs, sneezes, or touches their nose/skin or any surface other than the one they are working on.
- Only paper towels should be used in kitchens to dry the hands.
- Hand-washing with soap and hot water is generally adequate for infection control purposes.

Maintenance of equipment

- Routine functional inspection of commercial refrigerators and regular maintenance of food preparation equipment is necessary to prevent potential contamination of food.
- Care should be taken to use only chlorinated water or water from an accepted, uncontaminated water source during food preparation and in refrigerators and freezing equipment.
- All equipment (cutlery, crockery and food mixing containers) and work areas must be kept immaculately clean at all times.

Serving of food

- Food servers should be trained and closely supervised.
- Staff who are ill should not serve food.
- Special precautions should be taken to prevent direct manual contact with food. This includes no random touching, smelling or handling of food by anyone other than the patient being served.

- Suitable serving utensils must be used to minimise handling of the food.
- Open food or drink placed on display should be protected from contamination by consumers or dust and airborne micro-organisms with special containers or display cases.
- Portions of unconsumed food must not be served to another person but must be disposed of.
- If plastic gloves are worn to prevent food contamination, they should be replaced regularly and the hands washed to prevent contamination due to perspiration build-up inside the gloves.
- Leftover food should not be left indefinitely at the patient's bedside. If the patient has finished eating, unconsumed food should be removed for storage or disposal.
- Food waste should be removed from the patient-care area in covered containers and safely stored until sanitary disposal can be ensured.
- Baby feeds are especially at risk from contamination and resultant infection. High standards of hygiene, and extreme care in the preparation, handling and decanting of milk feeds are essential for safe consumption.
- Feeds should be mixed and refrigerated as soon as possible.
- Mixing bowls and other equipment must preferably be steam-sterilised or boiled daily.
- Only dedicated jugs and boiling water should be used for warming feeds in hospitals.
- Particular care should be taken when washing babies' bottles:
  - wash the bottle and teat separately in an anionic detergent
  - rinse and sterilise by autoclaving, or
  - disinfect by pasteurisation (boiling) in hot water.
- Feeding bottles should not be handled unnecessarily. Mothers should be shown hygienic care for feeding bottles and taught that unconsumed milk must be measured and disposed of, not kept for a later feed.

Pest control

- Pests such as flies and rodents may transmit salmonella. Regular pest control is therefore essential in storerooms and kitchens.
- Leftover food must be safely disposed of to prevent attracting pests and rodents.
- Most pesticides are contact poison and must remain on surfaces long enough for all insects to have contact with them – cleaning staff should take this into account: cleaning must be done before spraying and not repeated for at least 24–48 hours.
- In kitchens the floor can be sprayed, but insect bait and gels work better, due to the necessity of cleaning work surfaces before use.
- Rodents (rats and mice) often live in sewers and travel into the kitchens through sink outlets with broken or absent grease traps. Where there are rodents, cats soon follow.
- Ants may carry salmonella, proteus or clostridium as well as enteric pathogens such as escherichia and klebsiella.

Linen management

Used linen plays a limited but important role in infection control. Contaminated linen poses the risk of transmitting micro-organisms, of which some will act as opportunistic pathogens under the right conditions. Laundry staff are exposed to conditions such as childhood ailments (e.g. chickenpox), hepatitis A, salmonellosis and fungal diseases. Faecal contamination of linen is a common occurrence and carries the highest risk of transmitting pathogens as the organic material protects the microbes from dying due to dehydration.

Many institutions advocate the soaking of contaminated and soiled linen in disinfectant solutions as a means of infection control. This is totally unacceptable as disinfectants are deactivated by organic matter and soap. This includes often-used chemical compounds such as sodium hypochlorite, chlorine and quaternary ammonium compounds. Washing and pasteurising with hot water, tumble-drying and ironing is a cheaper and more efficient infection control measure. Incomplete disinfection may promote unsafe laundry handling and subsequent transmission of pathogens to laundry staff.

Definitions

Used linen is linen that has been in contact with a patient or a work surface even though it might not be visibly soiled.

Soiled linen is visibly dirty linen, containing organic matter, body fluids such as blood, or any other foreign substances perceived to be unclean.

Contaminated linen need not be visibly soiled but is linen that has been in contact with a patient or surface and carries a higher than acceptable load of confirmed/possible pathogens such as viruses from an incontinent patient with hepatitis B, smallpox or anthrax spores. Hospital linen generally contains a biological load of ± 70% Gram-negative bacilli, such as *Eschericia coli* and *Pseudomonas aeruginosa* and ± 20% Gram-positive cocci, such as *Staphylococcus aureus.*

Infested linen contains living/viable parasites such as scabies, lice or their nits.

Principles of linen management

Specifications for used-laundry bags

The bags should be waterproof or impermeable, strong and tear-resistant, lightweight, washable and relatively cheap to replace. Two types of soluble laundry bags are available:

- Warm-water-soluble bags, which are expensive, but may be indicated for the transport of highly contagious linen such as that of patients with viral haemorrhagic fevers, extreme weeping dermatitis or extensive septic open wounds. The bag dissolves at a relatively high temperature, preventing it from weakening due to possible damp contents.
- Cold-water-soluble bags are at risk of disintegrating from excessively wet contents, causing environmental contamination and staff exposure. Some bags have a cold-water soluble seal whilst the rest of the bag is insoluble to prevent accidental spillage of the contents.

Ordinary plastic bags may be used inside an outer canvas bag for the safe transportation of laundry. Colour-coding opaque bags to indicate the destination of the bag and/or the exposure risk is an effective way of warning illiterate laundry handlers of possible danger. Impermeable laundry bags avoid the risk of attracting pests such as flies, ants and cockroaches as well as cats, mice and dogs.

Sorting used linen

- Linen is sorted in the patient-care area where it is produced and must never be carried from one point to another before discarding.
- The used-linen container should be at hand, placed at the bedside so that folded linen can be put directly into it, after ensuring that there are no foreign objects such as clothing, linen savers or waterproof sheets inside.
- Used linen should never be shaken out, as this spreads contaminating micro-organisms over the direct environment, the handlers' clothing and hands. The surrounding air should be disturbed as little as possible, to contain possible contamination.
- Used linen should not be sorted again and should be handled as little as possible.
- The filled linen container should be sealed and stored separately from the clean linen supply. If plastic bags are used, the bags

must be sealed when they are three-quarters full. Staples should not be used as these perforate the bags.

- Less-soiled linen should be separated from more heavily soiled pieces as the latter may stain and further contaminate the former.
- Curtains should never be washed with bed linen. Curtains are generally washed less frequently and any microbial contamination transmitted from bed linen to the curtains would remain on these surfaces for longer periods.
- Soiled linen such as babies' nappies or bloodsoaked linen from casualty, theatre or maternity rooms is considered contaminated and must be placed in waterproof containers such as colour-coded (yellow) plastic bags to identify the contents. Exposure to this type of used linen poses a high risk of infection to handlers and the linen must be removed and laundered as soon as possible. Heavily contaminated linen should be double-bagged if the plastic bags are thin and likely to tear.
- Linen from patients with known highly contagious diseases, such as haemorrhagic fever (with bleeding) or anthrax, must be double-bagged in plastic before being placed in paper bag(s) or cardboard boxes, then steam-autoclaved and/or incinerated.
- Laundry handlers must wash their hands after touching used linen as it contains a cross-selection of all the micro-organisms from the resident patients, staff and the environment. The linen from deceased patients will contain all the micro-organisms the patient harboured whilst alive.
- The linen of patients in intensive care units should be changed six-hourly in order to minimise the contaminating bioburden on the bed.

Transporting laundry

- Filled laundry bags must be removed from patient-care areas as soon as possible to avoid leakage and environmental contamination.
- Bags must always be carefully lifted and placed onto a trolley or other means of conveyance. Bags that are dragged along the floor might tear or leave a track of contamination. If bags are thrown they may burst or contaminating aerosols may be forced through the material of the bag. The trolley must be washed with detergent and hot water after all the used linen has been unloaded, and dried carefully before any clean linen bags can be placed on it.
- Canvas or material laundry bags must be used only once before washing.
- No workers must be allowed to sit, lie or sleep on top of bags of used linen, especially if the bags are permeable or have been soiled by the contents inside.
- Laundry staff must wear gloves and waterproof aprons or impermeable gowns when handling used linen. Any lesions on their hands must be covered with waterproof dressings and any suspected occupational disease or exposure to infection should immediately be reported to a supervisor.
- Special storage areas should be available to store used laundry. These areas should be hygienic, dry, weatherproof and burglar-proof and separate from the main work area.

Rinsing/sluicing laundry: in-house

- Soiled linen should be machine-rinsed, using a cold cycle before being washed at a temperature of at least 90°C (194°F).
- All used linen should be sorted at least once at the bedside or the place where it was used, before being packed into canvas/nylon laundry bags.
- Contaminated linen must be sorted twice, using the following procedure:
  - The staff in the patient care area/the place it was produced sort it the first time.
  - Linen that is damp, wet, or visibly soiled must be placed in colour-coded (e.g. yellow) plastic bags that are marked with

the number of the ward and contents.

- Towels must be counted separately, packed and marked for each patient care area, as they are usually required again quickly.
- Linen heavily soiled with blood, infested with parasites such as lice, contaminated by a patient with freely exuding wounds, or used by a patient with a contact-transmissible condition, must be placed in a colour-coded plastic bag, which must be additionally marked with a biohazard warning sticker and sealed to warn the sluicing staff of the possibility of infection.
- The coloured bags can then be stored with the other bags containing used linen to be transported to the sluicing facility in the laundry room.
- The coloured plastic bags are torn open at the sluicing facility and the contents carefully sorted a second time before being placed one item at a time into the sluicing machine. Foreign objects such as patients' clothing, personal possessions or linen savers should be removed and sent back or discarded in medical waste containers.
- The sluicing machine(s) should rinse the linen with cold water and a chemical additive. The run-off water will be drained into the hospital's sewage system. External laundry services: after tumble-drying, the damp sluiced linen should be packed into transparent plastic bags to distinguish it from unsluiced washing. These bags can then be placed in a canvas/nylon laundry bag. A prepared label that specifies the contents (and number of items) must be tied to the bag
- In-house laundry services: After rinsing, the linen can be washed as normal.
- Each laundry trolley should be washed with soap and water before a new canvas/nylon laundry bag is placed in it.

- The staff of the sluicing facility must wear boots, caps, dust-proof or high-particulate filter face masks, gloves and plastic aprons to protect themselves from contamination and soiling.
- The linen bag handlers may wear their ordinary clothing due to the use of impermeable plastic bags for contaminated linen.
- No item of soiled linen should be hand-rinsed/sluiced in a patient-care area as this leads to contamination of the environment and the real risk of transmitting infection. If rinsing/sluicing has to be done, a washing machine should be used and the work area should be separate from the general patient-care areas.
- 'Spot cleaning' or hand rinsing/sluicing will spread a small spot of soiling/contamination over the rest of the wet item, giving the previously contained micro-organisms access to the whole item for further growth if it is not washed promptly with detergent. If such a piece of laundry is left in the patient-care area, spillage, environmental contamination and exposure of the patients and staff to pathogens is likely.
- Soiled linen containing solid organic matter such as stool should carefully be emptied into a flush toilet or sluice bowl. Solid matter will contaminate the washing machine and the rest of the laundry.

Laundering linen

- The process of washing linen as a method of disinfecting requires that temperatures of between 65°C (150°F) and 93°C (200°F) be maintained for 10–25 minutes in a fully laden machine. Mixing times of 4–8 minutes must be allowed to ensure that the load is completely penetrated by the chemicals and hot water.
- Washing reduces the total organism count on used linen due to the mechanical movement, detergent and chemical interaction,

dilution of the microbial concentration and drainage of contaminated water.

- Soiled linen that has come into contact with infectious diseases (such as hepatitis B/C and the human immunosuppressive virus), should be transported to the laundry in waterproof bags. The bags must be opened directly into a washing machine and the unsorted contents washed at 90°C (194°F) with detergent and the necessary chemical additives. A temperature of 90°C (194°F) ensures pasteurisation, increasing the safety level of the clean linen.
- Infested linen should be handled like any other contaminated linen and washed at 90°C (194°F) to kill the contents. It need not be autoclaved or boiled beforehand.
- Bundled or rolled linen must be untangled before washing. Detergents, hot water and chemicals cannot penetrate deep enough into the load if this is not done, leaving the centre of the supposedly washed contents still contaminated, infectious and unusable.
- Open-air or tumble-drying and ironing completes the pasteurisation of the washed linen.

Handling clean linen

- Just after washing, the microbiological load of linen is at its lowest level. Subsequent handling dictates the future levels.
- Clean vehicles, trolleys or other conveyances must be used to transport clean linen, preferably packed in plastic sheaths or impermeable bags. This keeps the linen dust-free and clean till it reaches the patient-care areas.
- Storage areas should be clean, dry, dust-free and access-restricted, to avoid accidental contamination. No patient or untrained person should handle clean linen as this increases the microbial load on the outer layers.

- Linen placed on any other patient's bed, or which has dropped on the floor, should be discarded as contaminated and rewashed.
- Autoclaving clean linen is unnecessary, except under extreme circumstances, e.g. for patients with extensive burn wounds or immunosuppression due to bone marrow transplants. Uncontaminated clean linen is safe for all other patients.
- Laundry staff should be aware of safe hand hygiene practices and avoid handling clean linen if they are sick.

Waste management

Most healthcare facilities produce medical waste at an alarming rate. The current tendency to use single-use sterile packs and labour-saving disposables increases the amount of medical waste. Plastic disposables are difficult to degrade cleanly, even by incineration.

The question that healthcare facilities should be asking is how to avoid producing waste rather than trying to find the easiest disposal method. If the source can be controlled or eliminated, the impact on hospitals, other healthcare facilities and the environment will be smaller. Collection and disposal of medical waste can be extremely expensive if it is done correctly. In local communities, many people live on waste dumps and make a precarious living retrieving items thought to be re-usable. In the process they are extensively exposed to household and medical waste and all the opportunistic pathogens proliferating there.

Classifying waste

Medical waste – also called clinical or hospital waste – consists of human and animal tissue, blood, drugs, swabs, syringes and non-toxic items, such as household rubbish and waste from hospital kitchens and maintenance workshops. In actual fact, only part of the waste is infectious and a risk to handlers, patients and the community at large. To consider all medical waste infectious has serious cost implications for disposal and has no scientific basis. By isolating the infectious (biohazardous) component, the volume of medical waste can be reduced. Only this portion of medical waste (which is detailed below) should receive special attention.

Blood and body fluids

As a standard precaution, this includes everything that has been in contact with the patient's blood, tissues or body fluids. Barrier precautions are employed to prevent exposure via the mucous membranes or skin to infective body materials. This form of waste includes wound dressings, contaminated disposable items, soiled surgical drapes, swabs and bandages, disposable urine and sputum bottles, paper soaked with nasal or throat secretions, tongue depressors, baby napkins, wound drainage from patient care areas, etc.

The CDC makes specific mention of the following waste in long-term care facilities:

- blood-soiled items, dressings, etc. from all residents
- incontinence pads and other items soiled with faeces from residents known to have salmonella, shigella, or hepatitis A
- sharps which have punctured or cut human skin from any resident or which have been contaminated and are in need of disposal.

Healthcare workers, patients and waste handlers are at greatest risk of infection from this source.

Microbiological waste

This consists of blood and other tissues/body substances such as faeces, cultures and other laboratory specimens, contaminated test tubes, pipettes, capillary tubes and disposable equipment. This form of waste is usually considered infectious because of heavy concen-

trations of organisms in the culture mediums. At greatest risk of infection from this source are the laboratory staff and the waste and specimen handlers.

Sharp objects ('sharps')

These are items such as needles and syringes, scalpel blades, glass items, empty ampoules and vials, discarded test tubes, staples, lancets, caps from infusion sets as well as the metal parts of intravenous infusion devices, etc. At greatest risk of infection from this source are staff members caring for patients, waste handlers and the community at large.

Pathological waste

This consists of items such as stillborn foetuses, amputated limbs, bone and dissected tissue, expired drugs and pharmaceutical products, human excreta and secreta, human waste from surgical theatres and laboratories, heavy metals (mercury, aluminum, silver) contained in X-ray development fluid, cytotoxic drugs and radioisotopes.

Exposure risk depends on the type of waste and the volume. What was infectious during life usually remains so after death. Pathogenic organisms may be present in solid hospital waste in high concentrations – especially in the presence of organic substances (e.g. human tissue or body fluids). Paper and cotton fabric (such as swabs) may harbour active viruses for between 5–8 days.

Household (non-infectious/non-clinical) waste

This consists of items such as plastic/paper wrappers, disposable plates, containers and cups, paper towels, boxes, tins, empty aerosol and aluminum cans, kitchen waste (peels and vegetable matter), discarded food and office waste that holds no infection risk for patients, staff members or the community.

Collecting and transporting infectious waste

Waste management aims to protect the facility's staff, patients, visitors and the external community against contamination, soiling, loose waste and spills. The minimal exposure of waste handlers during all stages of waste handling is important. Appointing a waste control manager and team may be cost-effective in the long run.

Sorting waste at the production point means that infectious waste is placed directly into the appropriate container and need not be handled again. All waste containers must be strong enough and large enough to contain the waste without tearing, rupturing or collapsing. Plastic bags usually need to be at least 30–45 microns thick to be safe. On average, waste-filled plastic bags are picked up and moved at least 6–8 times on their way to the incinerator, risking damage to the bags and exposure of the waste handler or porter to infection or injury.

Double-bagging waste: Double-bagging means placing a sealed bag, knotted end down, into another plastic bag before sealing the second one as well. Double-bagging highly infectious waste may be necessary in high-risk areas such as P4 isolation wards with blood-borne infectious patients; in hospitals with a high level of hospital-acquired (nosocomial) infections or acute in-patient services such as paediatrics. Research shows that there is no aseptic advantage in double-bagging all potentially contaminated items from general isolation rooms or clinical laboratories. Using **single, heavy-duty plastic bags** may be more economical than using double, lighter-weight bags for the transport of infectious waste.

Sharps: Microwaving, autoclaving or incinerating and burying the residue of sharps containers in a landfill dump are ideal disposal methods.

Solid waste: Solid infectious waste should ideally be collected in colour-coded plastic bags, transported, microwaved, incinerated or steam-autoclaved and then disposed of in a sanitary landfill (dump). The following items are classified as solid waste:

- Blood-soaked disposables are discarded into colour-coded plastic bags before transportation to the incinerator/autoclave. Items should be pre-rinsed in case the container bursts, causing blood splashes which will harden inside the autoclave.
- In a clinic/at home: contaminated items can be saturated with bleach (1 part bleach and 9 parts luke-warm water) for 20–30 minutes, drained, sealed and placed in a secure area until disposal.
- Chemical disinfection should never be used on solid waste because of the problem of penetration – not all pathogens will be reached by the disinfectant.
- Microbiological and pathological waste should always be steam-autoclaved and then buried or incinerated.

Fluid waste: Consists of bulk blood, aspirated fluids, secretions and excretions that should be carefully poured down a drain connected to a sanitary sewer. Everything that can be safely disposed of down a flush sluice or toilet should be disposed of in this way, as it is mixed with the general sewage and decontaminated in the process.

General waste disposal methods

No single treatment technique is ideal for all types of waste. Several disposal methods for infectious waste exist, which are explained below.

Incineration

Incineration is a very popular and safe disposal method (if the rules are followed!). In theory, incineration can dispose of all combustible waste. In practice the opposite is true. Old, poorly designed or inefficient hospital incinerators cannot destroy all pathogens and viruses at temperatures below 1000°C. Modern multi-chamber pathological waste incinerators need to be built to withstand temperatures of 1000–1500°C throughout the incinerator, completely vapourising effluent, gas and smoke, while reducing the toxicity of the emissions. Infectious waste should only be burnt at a minimum of 1000°C.

The following are some of the general problems associated with incineration:

- Air pollution is caused by the smoke, ash emissions and hydrochloric acid (the basis of 'acid rain') resulting from the combustion of polyvinyl chloride plastics.
- Sharps and pathogenic waste may not be completely destroyed.
- Carcinogenic gases are formed by incomplete combustion of some plastics and all cytotoxic drugs.
- Residual waste may cause blockage of the furnace.
- Incineration may become an expensive method of disposal in the long term.

Land-filling ('dumping')

This is a very popular and cheap method of disposal but is not safe unless well planned, managed and supervised in a sanitary landfill site. Uncontrolled dumping is hazardous to the community at large as people live and work on landfills, reclaiming and recycling waste (scavenging). Incoming medical waste should be transported in plastic bags that are immediately torn open to encourage decomposition in a designated area of the landfill. The contents must be covered immediately with at least 80 cm of soil and rock. It is relatively far safer to bury compressed waste in a landfill, as all fluid has been expressed and the rest made unidentifiable/irretrievable.

The following are some of the general problems associated with dumping:

- Exposure to infection readily occurs at the disposal site due to direct contact between refuse workers/scavengers and the waste.
- Water pollution may occur via runoff or leaching.
- Scavengers may salvage contaminated or radio-active articles.
- Disposable babies' nappies or adult incontinence napkins/sheaths are a source of enteric viruses that may survive in waste for as long as 7–10 days.
- Methane gas produced by decomposing waste is toxic and may cause death in extreme cases.
- Biological vectors such as flies, ants and cockroaches breed on refuse heaps and may spread disease.

Steam-autoclaving

This is widely used, because it is a reliable and easily controlled process. The waste does not need to be sterile, as changing the biological character of it reduces/eliminates the potential to cause disease and reduces the microbial load contained in it.

The following are some general problems associated with this method:

- Containers for the waste must be large enough and permeable for the steam to penetrate and condense on the contents.
- Separate autoclaves are needed for preparing items for sterile procedures and for waste management.
- Trained staff and good supervision are required.
- Each load needs to be biologically monitored to ensure safety (a spore culture done).
- Steam processes can be expensive and time-consuming as only relatively small volumes of waste can be handled at any given time.
- Land-filling or alternative disposal of the residue is still required as there is no guarantee of steam penetrating to the core of the load.

Microwaving

This type of technology is gaining ground in areas where incineration of waste is not readily accepted any more. The disposal unit usually shreds the waste in a controlled environment before wetting it and then treating it with microwaves. Microwaves heat the waste from the inside (unlike other thermal treatments, which heat externally), destroying micro-organisms by the steam that is generated in the process. The heat temperatures are the same as for autoclaving waste, and the process is monitored by using microbiological spore test indicators, again as in any autoclaving process. The end result is sterilised waste products which can be discharged in a biohazardous solid-waste landfill site. The only products for which this system is not recommended are pathological wastes such as human tissue, blood and foetal matter. Medical waste is usually made unrecognisable and irretrievable and therefore safe after the process. Some general problems associated with this method are that health, pollution and noise risks can be caused by maintenance of the shredder component of the system: waste can jam or break the hammer grinder, or staff may be exposed to aerosolised particles containing pathogens or volatised chemicals during loading, cleaning or maintenance of equipment.

Disposal into sewage systems

Waste can usually be disposed of into sewage systems if the healthcare facility has access to a modern sanitary sewer system and/or a large sewage treatment plant. Fluid waste can be flushed as noted (refer to page 154). Solid medical waste is more difficult to dispose of as the parts have to be broken up and ground finer in order to flush it successfully.

Some general problems associated with this method of disposal are:

- The format of pathogenic waste is changed, but the pathogens themselves are not affected.
- Sufficient grinding units, as well as large supplies of water and electricity are needed.

- The volume of waste is greatly increased.
- The smell and noise level may be unacceptable.
- Soft materials such as rubber and plastic are difficult to grind.
- The possibility of creating hazardous aerosols is a risk to workers and the environment.

Developing an effective infectious waste control programme

It is short-sighted if a hospital does not have an infectious-waste control programme. Aspects of the topic that have to be addressed include policy on:

- What waste is considered infective.
- The use of special containers for infectious waste.
- Waste collection and movement within the facility.
- Storage conditions.
- Treatment procedures (e.g. steam autoclaving).
- Emergency procedures for containment and clean-up of hazardous material spills.
- Shipment of untreated infectious waste from the hospital for disposal.
- The loading and unloading, washing (and disinfecting where indicated in abnormal situations) of transport trucks.
- Record keeping.
- Employee training, education and counselling.
- Occupational health programmes for prophylactic immunisation, care of in-service exposure (especially for those workers with needle-prick injuries and those who handle the incinerator, as many of the resultant gases are toxic or carcinogenic) and injuries.

General considerations

- Waste handlers must be informed if the waste contains potentially infectious material or agents. Ideally their procedures should be of such a standard that special warnings are unnecessary – as with all healthcare practices. Unfortunately this seldom happens and it may be necessary to apply special biohazard stickers to the outside of the waste bags as a warning.

- Protective clothing such as impermeable gloves, overalls and face shields/masks should be provided as a matter of course to all waste handlers.
- Recycling uncontaminated waste such as glass, plastic, aluminum, tins, wood, paper and boxes, heavy metals from runoffs and water may help keep the environment safe as well as supplying an income to the facility. Up to 60% of household and unsoiled clinical waste can be retrieved and sold.
- Solid infectious waste should be stored in a safe (locked) area accessible only to staff involved with the disposal process.
- Safe transport of sealed impervious waste containers to the disposal area is one of the employer's primary responsibilities.

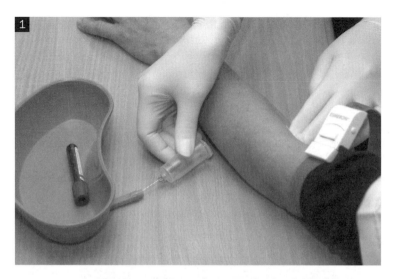

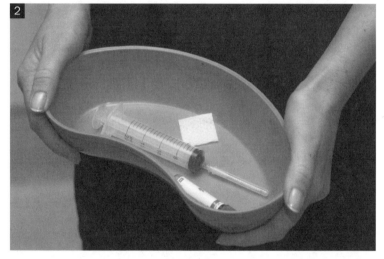

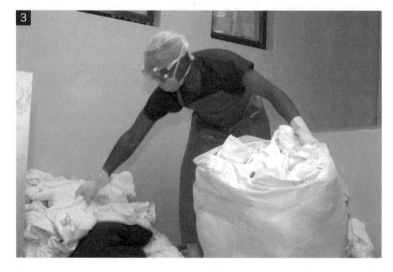

The international biohazard symbol

1 The cap of the vacuum tube is placed against a solid surface, the needle is inserted into it, hooked and lifted so that it slides downwards. This is a one-handed technique as the needle can now safely be unscrewed from the vacuum tube via the cap.

2 All sharps should be transported in a safety container and not carried open.

3 Sorting linen and counting items must take place under controlled circumstances in an area that is easily cleaned, by staff wearing the approprite protective clothing in relation to the risk of exposure.

4 Used needles and syringes should never be manipulated by hand, but rather discarded as a unit into a rigid, specially marked sharps disposal container.

5 Handwashing should take place using the correct technique, appropriate soap, under running water for the correct length of time. Paper towels should be used to dry hands well, before disposal.

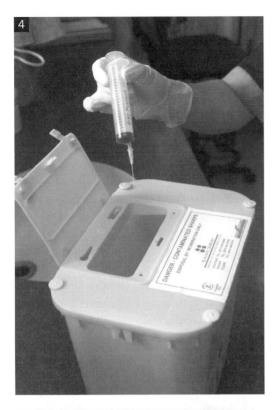

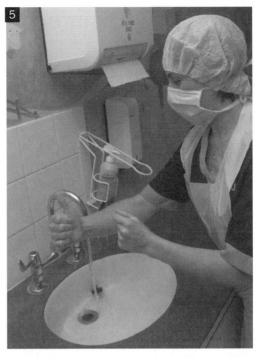

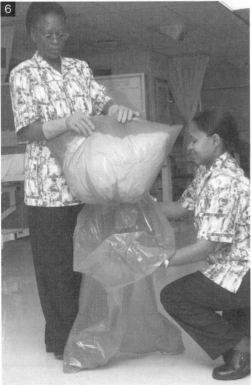

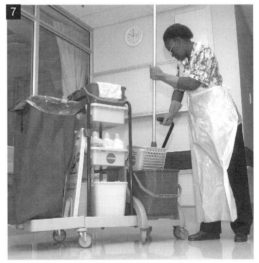

6 Double bagging medical waste in colour-coded bags: the filled bag is placed knotted end down into a second bag, which is held resting on the floor to prevent it slipping from the holder's grasp. The second bag is then knotted closed as well.

7 Well cared for and maintained cleaning equipment. All the necessary supplies and items are collected on the trolley by the cleaning staff member, who wears the correct protective gear in relation to the exposure risk.

5 | Disinfection and sterilisation

Disinfection

Disinfection is a step between the concepts of 'surgically clean' and 'sterile'. Many healthcare workers speak of an item or their hands as being 'sterile' when they really mean clean or disinfected. Disinfection does not imply sterility, but is a phase leading up to it. A wide continuum of results fall within the spectrum of 'disinfection', varying from low levels barely above cleanliness, to high levels a few micro-organisms away from sterility.

Definition. Disinfection is the inactivation or removal of vegetative micro-organisms but not necessarily bacterial spores from surfaces.

Levels of disinfection

Three levels of disinfection are generally accepted:
1. A high level where all vegetative (growing) and non-spore-forming micro-organisms are **destroyed**.
2. An intermediate level where all of the vegetative micro-organisms, excluding bacterial spores, are **inactivated**.
3. A low level where most of the vegetative micro-organisms, excluding some bacteria, bacterial spores, viruses and some fungi are **inactivated**.

In healthcare institutions disinfection is generally indicated for:
- pre-operative skin and tissue preparation
- preparation of hands before and after aseptic procedures are performed
- hand disinfection after casual contact with a patient or the patient-care environment

- decontamination of specific used/soiled instruments or equipment before cleaning (e.g. those used during skin-penetrating procedures on HIV-positive patients)
- terminal disinfection of contaminated patient-care areas after cleaning (e.g. isolation rooms)
- terminal disinfection of heat- or pressure-sensitive patient-care equipment or instruments after cleaning (e.g. endoscopes)
- care of cleaned equipment too large to fit into autoclaves (e.g. trolleys) before reuse.

Commonly used disinfection methods

Four methods are generally accepted.

Cleaning

This method is described in the section on 'General cleaning methods' in chapter 4, page 140.

Heat (Pasteurisation)

Economical and easy to use, either dry or in steam/fluid form. Most micro-organisms excluding heat-resistant bacterial spores are destroyed after twenty minutes of exposure to water at 65°C (150°F). The warmer the water, the quicker the process and the less time needed. The holding time starts as soon as the coldest part of the load has reached the required temperature.

Table 5.1: Pasteurisation schedule

Temperature	Disinfection (holding time)
65°C	10 minutes
70°C	05 minutes
80°C	01 minute
90°C	01 second

The prerequisites for pasteurisation are that:
- all items must be clean/washed and rinsed
- all air is removed from hollow instruments or tubes
- no new item can be added to a cycle that has already begun
- items emerge wet from the steam/water and must then be dried as only completely dry items are considered adequately disinfected.

Advantages: No chemical residue is left on surfaces, and equipment can be used as soon as it has dried. At home or in a clinic pasteurisation may be carried out by using water that has boiled and cooled to the required temperature in a covered pot on the stove or fire.

Disadvantage: The greatest disadvantage of heat is the potential damage to surfaces. Unless special machines are used, the process can be time-consuming and labour-intensive. As the wet items may be extremely hot, measures must be taken to prevent workers from burning themselves when handling pasteurised objects. Leaving the objects to cool in the boiled, closed container may be one way to achieve this.

Chemical disinfection:

The term 'chemical disinfectant' includes **antiseptics** which are disinfectants which can be used on living surfaces, such as the skin and tissues, without undue toxicity or damage, depending on the right concentration. **Germicides** are environmental disinfectants that will damage tissue and skin. In the proper concentrations and with the correct exposure time, these chemicals will sterilise surfaces.

The use of chemicals is unreliable and the process difficult to control. Inappropriately chosen or applied solutions increase costs and microbial resistance to disinfectants. The use of chemical disinfectants is indicated if no alternative method of disinfection is appropriate.

Some points to note:
- Disinfectants that are mixed with detergents or other chemicals in a bid to 'improve their activity' are soon deactivated or neutralised, especially sodium hypochlorite. Mixing and storage containers must therefore be manufactured from an appropriate material, otherwise the disinfectant is deactivated from the start.
- Fresh chemical solutions must be prepared daily, carefully measured and mixed before storing in an appropriate, clean/sterile container.
- Materials such as paper, cork, cotton, certain plastics, and organic matter (blood and body fluids/ tissue) weaken disinfectants. Weakened solutions may harbour micro-organisms and become an active, unknown source of infection.
- All items must be clean, dry and dust-free before disinfection, as extra water or organic matter dilutes, deactivates and neutralises chemical solutions. Cleaning reduces the microbial load on surfaces, allowing chemicals to function more efficiently.
- The appropriate concentration of chemicals is important as surfaces may be damaged by strong solutions. Weak solutions may not be germicidal, allowing micro-organisms to live and multiply in the solution. This is generally what happens if bottles of old (expired) or weakened disinfectants are topped up with a new supply. The micro-organisms become resistant to the chemical and the growing numbers neutralise the active ingredients. The 'disinfectant' now becomes an 'infectant'!

- All disinfectants are not equally effective against all types of micro-organisms, and do not have the same range of action:
  - quaternary ammonium compounds and chlorhexadine are mostly effective against Gram-positive cocci
  - 70% ethyl or 60% isopropyl alcohol is effective against most vegetative bacteria and enveloped viruses but not against bacterial spores
  - iodine and acetic acid are mostly effective against pseudomonas
  - hypochlorites and glutaraldehyde are more active against the hepatitis B and the human immunosuppressive virus than other disinfectants.
- Temperature plays a part in disinfection. Though room temperature is generally acceptable, slightly warmer solutions are usually more efficient. Beyond the ideal temperature, the activity of chemicals will be reduced.
- Disinfectants require the right exposure time in which to work efficiently. The weaker the solution and the greater the contamination or load of micro-organisms on a surface, the more time is needed. Only 70–90% alcohol, iodine or chlorine are able to disinfect non-living surfaces in a few seconds, though the use of more than 70% alcohol encourages micro-organisms to form spores. Generally, the longer the exposure, the better the results. When the active ingredient in the solution has evaporated, the chemical looses efficacy.

- Disinfectants kept in spray bottles are contaminated by the equivalent volume of air that is sucked in when a volume of the fluid is sprayed out. If the contents are not changed at least every 48 hours, micro-organisms start to grow in the solution, resulting in the deactivation of the active ingredients.
- Environmental disinfection is a controversial subject. General disinfection is expensive, corrosive to surfaces and labour-intensive. As pointed out in the previous section, disinfection should only be considered in high-risk patient-care areas or if contamination with contagious matter or human body fluid/blood has occurred. Usually, good hygiene and a high level of cleanliness will ensure a safe patient-care environment.
- Fumigation with formaldehyde vapour is sporocidal during prolonged exposure, but the vapour is unpleasant and toxic, has poor penetration and has to be neutralised after use. Surfaces must be clean beforehand as dust and organic matter will deactivate the drops of disinfectant. This process is seldom carried out today.
- At home the following may be used for disinfection: carbolic soap; household bleach (a freshly prepared solution of 1 part bleach to 9 parts cooled, boiled water); spirit vinegar (1 part spirit vinegar to 9 parts cooled, boiled water) or a saline solution (5 ml to 750 ml cooled boiled water) may safely be used to disinfect hands, wounds and washed surfaces.

Table 5.2: Schedule of general disinfectants

Disinfectant	Examples	Characteristics	Uses	Advantages	Disadvantages
Alcohol (70% v.v.)	▪ Alcohol ▪ Isopropyl alcohol ▪ Methylated spirits ▪ Ethyl alcohol	▪ Diluted with water to a 60-90% v/v solution, 70% works the best ▪ Active against most bacteria, but not effective against non-enveloped viruses/fungi/bacterial spores	▪ Skin disinfectant ▪ Disinfection of clean surfaces (non-living) ▪ Can be mixed with other chemicals (e.g. iodine) to form more effective compounds	▪ Quick action	▪ Highly flammable ▪ Toxic ▪ Evaporates quickly – contact time not always sufficient for all killing ▪ Corrodes some types of metal/rubber ▪ Does not penetrate organic matter
Aldehyde	▪ Formaldehyde (Formalin)	▪ Effective against bacteria, viruses, fungi, parasites and spores. ▪ Most vegetative bacteria are inactivated after 10 minutes. Exposure of 6–10 hours may be needed for sterilisation. ▪ 1–5% concentration of aqueous formalin is used as a preservative. ▪ Formaldehyde is often used as a gas	▪ Preserving tissue ▪ Fumigation of small areas ▪ Disinfection of clean equipment	▪ Dependable if used correctly ▪ A measure of activity is retained in the presence of small amounts of organic contamination ▪ Slight residual activity	▪ Very irritating to the skin, airways, eyes, mucosa ▪ Deactivated by moderate to high levels of organic material ▪ Long exposure times are required for disinfection ▪ Formaldehyde vapour has weak penetration (e.g. in tubes) ▪ Has to be washed off surfaces before reuse ▪ Neutralisation with ammonia may be necessary for some items

Disinfectant	Examples	Characteristics	Uses	Advantages	Disadvantages
	▪ Glutaraldehyde	▪ Glutaraldehyde is affected by pH ▪ Must be activated and buffered	▪ Disinfection/ sterilisation of endoscopes and heat-sensitive items ▪ Disinfection/ sterilisation of clean surfaces ▪ Useful when combined with surfactant as surface detergent/ disinfectant	▪ May be effective for 7–14 days if the directions for use are followed ▪ Non-staining, relatively non-corrosive	▪ Irritating to the eyes, airway, skin and mucosa ▪ Toxic ▪ Allergenic ▪ Must be rinsed with sterile water ▪ Deactivated by organic matter ▪ Long exposure times are required for sterilisation (3–10 hours) ▪ Expensive ▪ Can be corrosive
Chlorhexidine	▪ Hand disinfectants, antiseptic soap, hand- and gynaecological creams e.g. handwashing soap, etc.	▪ Only for use on living tissues (not the environment/instruments) ▪ 70% alcohol increases the bactericidal speed ▪ Ineffective against mycobacteria, spores, fungi and viruses	▪ Active against some Gram-positive and -negative organisms ▪ Preservative in pharmacological preparations	▪ Relatively non-irritating disinfectant for the skin and some mucosal areas (excluding the eyes and ears)	▪ Easily deactivated by organic material and other chemicals (as well as cork, soap and some plastics) ▪ Must remain in contact with surfaces for at least 5 minutes ▪ Hard/alkaline water will cause precipitation of active ingredients needed for disinfection ▪ Microbes attain resistance with relative ease

Disinfectant	Examples	Characteristics	Uses	Advantages	Disadvantages
					▪ Short shelf life in aqueous solutions (7 days) ▪ Not effective against pseudomonas species ▪ May cause deafness if it penetrates the middle ear
Halogens	▪ Hypochlorite ▪ Chlorine ▪ Dyes, e.g. 'Chrystal Violet', 'Brilliant Green', 'Methyl Blue'	▪ Active against bacteria, fungi, viruses, some spores ▪ Releases active chlorine, measured in parts per million (ppm). ▪ At least 250–10 000 ppm free chlorine is usually required for disinfection. ▪ pH is a critical factor and has to be correct	▪ Effective for disinfecting clean instruments, equipment and surfaces – must remain in contact with surfaces for several minutes ▪ Hypochlorite is used for feeding bottles, general environmental disinfection, instruments and living tissues ▪ Dyes are used to colour compounds	▪ Ease of use ▪ Reasonably non-toxic ▪ Dyes are bactericidal and fungicidal ▪ Has a deodorising effect	▪ Easily deactivated by organic matter ▪ Irritating to eyes, skin and mucosa ▪ Corrodes metals and deteriorates fabrics ▪ Only fresh solutions made up daily in clean containers are dependable ▪ Chlorine granules have to be activated with fluid (water) and complete solution is necessary ▪ Chlorine evaporates quickly and the chlorine contents of compounds diminish progressively

Disinfectant	Examples	Characteristics	Uses	Advantages	Disadvantages
	▪ Iodine, e.g. 'Iodine Tincture' alcohol ▪ Iodiophor (iodine with a carrier)	▪ Iodine has a similar action to chlorine but evaporates more slowly	▪ Effective against fungi, bacteria, viruses and some spores	▪ Iodiophors are staining, non-irritating and are effective as long as the solution stays coloured ▪ Buffered iodine has low tissue toxicity ▪ Kills immediately, highly reactive ▪ Tuberculocidal, with extended contact time ▪ Not affected by hard water	▪ Allergenic (especially iodine) – has to be washed off the skin ▪ Inactivated by organic matter, must be applied multiple times to achieve disinfection ▪ Iodine may cause skin blistering when combined with alcohol for example
Phenol	▪ Carbolic acid ▪ Clear soluble phenol solutions, e.g. 'White phenol' ▪ Hexachlorophene e.g. 'Glyco-Thymol'	▪ White phenol is active against staphylococci, mycobacteria, and Gram-negative bacteria such as pseudomonas ▪ Incompatible with soap and detergents ▪ Hexachlorophene is relatively inactive against Gram-negative bacteria	▪ Disinfection of clean environmental surfaces ▪ Carbolic soap is used for soiled linen ▪ Adult staphylococci carriers: 10 days uninterrupted use without combining it with soap ▪ Disinfection of drains, floors, bedding, instruments ▪ Phenol is a preservative in pharmacological preparations	▪ Reasonably stable against deactivation if the concentration is accurate ▪ Active in acid conditions ▪ Active against some staphylococci and Gram-positive organisms ▪ Refined phenol can be used on living tissues ▪ Sporicidal	▪ Easily deactivated by organic matter, soap and plastic ▪ Unpleasant odour ▪ Less effective if diluted ▪ Undiluted phenol is corrosive ▪ Hexachlorophene is toxic to the central nervous system ▪ Effectiveness reduced by alkaline pH ▪ Toxicity increases cumulatively if absorbed through the skin

Disinfectant	Examples	Characteristics	Uses	Advantages	Disadvantages
Quaternary ammonia compounds ('QACs'/'QUATS')	▪ Cetrimide ▪ Benzalconium chloride (in some eye drops)	▪ Effective against staphylococci and other Gram-positive bacteria ▪ Ineffective against pseudomonas – easily grows in cetrimide ▪ Releases nitrogen and phosphorous from cells	▪ Cetrimide can be combined with chlorhexidine ▪ Seldom used singly	▪ Deodorising ▪ Often combined with detergent to loosen contamination ▪ Rapid action, non-toxic, colourless, stable, odourless ▪ Can be used in food preparation	▪ Easily deactivated by organic matter and soap ▪ Adsorption onto cotton and some plastics makes these compounds undependable ▪ Does not eliminate spores, TB, bacteria, some viruses
Oxidising agents	▪ Hydrogen peroxide	▪ Good effect against anaerobic bacteria	▪ Good for cleaning surgical site surfaces after closure ▪ Sterilising agent	▪ Moderately corrosive and limited toxicity ▪ Good environmental cleaning and deodorising agent	▪ Not very effective against viruses; bacterial and fungal spores unless combined with other agents ▪ Damaging to tissues, inhibits granulation and prolongs healing time ▪ Poor residual effect ▪ Deactivated by organic matter

Sterilisation

Sterilisation is the gold standard of all infection prevention and control methods, as it destroys al possible biohazardous material, leaving surfaces totally clear of all possibility of cross-infection. Many of the procedures used in healthcare settings aim at sterility, but there are specific requirements for this standard to be achieved, as discussed in this section. **Definition.** Sterilisation is the total eradication of all living micro-organisms and spores.

Commonly used sterilisation methods

Saturated steam under pressure

Steam under pressure is an efficient, non-toxic, economical and rapid sterilisation method if used correctly, as it kills micro-organisms by coagulating their protoplasm. This is the method of choice for all instruments that can withstand the moist heat of saturated steam under pressure, without deterioration or damage.

Sterilisation is dependent on temperature, time and pressure.

Table 5.3: Steam sterilisation schedule (The air extraction and drying required by an autoclave will extend the total time necessary for sterilisation).

Temperature	Sterilisation	Pressure (holding time)
121°C	15 minutes	15 kPa
126°C	10 minutes	20 kPa
134°C	03 minutes	30 kPa

- Air is removed by vacuum from the autoclave to speed up the process. The presence of air in the chamber reduces the steam pressure. As steam must penetrate to the core of the load, factors such as air removal, packaging material, arrangement of items inside the pack and the way packs are loaded are critical to the process.

- Maintenance, inspection and daily pre-work checking are essential to ensure the sterility of critical patient care equipment such as instruments. Autoclave monitoring methods include:
  - sensitive paper or adhesive tape strips that discolour when exposed to pressure and heat (placed inside or on the outer pack)
  - commercial paper tabs (placed inside all packs) that discolour when the heat, vacuum, load and humidity inside the autoclave chamber are correct
  - special sensitive tubes that melt when exposed to the correct high temperatures (placed in one load daily)
  - sealed biological test tubes containing bacterial spores that are incubated to monitor growth after sterilisation (placed in one load daily).
- The sterility of an autoclaved item only lasts until the moment the contents have been exposed to air or handling.
- One disadvantage of steam is that it does not penetrate anhydrous materials such as oils, greases and powders.
- At home or in a clinic, an ordinary pressure cooker may be utilised as an autoclave, or an item can be steamed in a microwave oven.

Dry heat

- Dry heat penetrates less efficiently and is less effective than moist heat.
- Dry heat may be used for heat-resistant instruments and glass, cutting-edge instruments, special needles, powders, oils and creams.
- Dry heat kills the micro-organisms by oxidising their protoplasm.
- At home or in a clinic the stove's oven may be utilised.
- Microwave ovens are not suitable for dry heat sterilisation.
- Higher temperatures, a longer heating-up time and longer exposure to the heat (holding time) are required for sterilisation.

Table 5.4: Dry heat schedule

Temperature	Sterilisation time
160°C	60 minutes
180°C	30 minutes

Disadvantages

- The process may require hours to complete, depending on the contents and size of the load.
- Heat distortion can occur, lubricants may dry out and many materials may become brittle or scorched.

Chemical sterilisation

Chemical sterilisation utilises gas such as ethylene oxide (EtO), and fluids, such as a formaldehyde and alcohol solution (see below for more examples).

Gas

Ethylene oxide gas (EtO) kills micro-organisms by permanently interfering with their metabolism. A special autoclave is needed to control the gas concentration, humidity, time, pressure and temperature required for the process. The autoclave must be situated separately from the general work area in a well-ventilated environment equipped with environmental gas monitors.

EtO may be used for intricate, delicate and heat-sensitive instruments and equipment (articulated and lensed endoscopes, electric cords and electrodes), plastic goods (catheters and heart pacemakers), unwashable pillows and soft toys.

To check the sterility of items, micro-biological controls as well as pressure-chemical-sensitive plastic, paper or adhesive tape strips may be used, inside or on the outer packs.

Disadvantages

- Gas sterilisation is time-consuming, expensive and risky.

- EtO is potentially toxic, mutagenous and carcinogenic. Staff members must be trained and well supervised to handle this sterilisation method. Minimal exposure time of the worker to the gas after the sterilisation cycle has been completed is important.
- Residual gas must be allowed to diffuse completely from items before use, as burns can be caused by contact of residual gas with tissue.
- All-metal or all-glass items can be used without aeration time, except for the time required for the packaging material to diffuse the gas.
- Soft materials such as plastic, rubber, vinyl and leather may retain the gas for several days at room temperature, even after processing in an aeration cabinet at elevated temperatures.

Table 5.5: Schedule of aeration time

Temperature	Aeration time after sterilisation
60°C	8 hours
40–49°C	12 hours

Fluid or 'cold' sterilisation

Chemical sterilisation is the least efficient or reliable method and should only be used if no alternative method is appropriate. Human error can compromise the process, e.g. by contaminating the sterilant or allowing it to evaporate or expire. Examples of chemical sterilants include:

- Formaldehyde (8%) and alcohol (70%) solutions
- Aqueous formalin (20%)
- Activated glutaraldehyde (2% aq.)
- Hydrogen peroxide
- Peracetic acid.

Chemical sterilisation is used for heat- and pressure-sensitive equipment, instruments and machines such as bronchoscopes, haemodialysis machines and operating microscopes. However, unless the process is carried properly and all the prerequisites are allowed, chemical 'sterilisation' only attains differing levels of disinfection. Cleaning, disinfection and sterilising are part of a single continuum with time allowance being the main influence, so short disinfecting times will not guarantee total sterility, but only attain a level of disinfection. High concentrations and prolonged exposure times of between six to ten hours are traditionally necessary for sterilisation.

Factors affecting chemical sterilisation include the freshness of the solution, the material from which the chemical container is manufactured, the cleanliness of the item placed in the chemical, total immersion and the amount of rinsing water or air that is trapped in a hollow instrument. Grease, dust or soil, organic matter, coagulated protein and even a layer of air can prevent the fluid from coming into contact with the microorganisms contaminating surfaces.

Disadvantages

- Like EtO, most chemicals are toxic and must be removed by rinsing or washing the item before it can be used.
- Many of the fluids are corrosive to metal, rubber and plastic.
- Inappropriate and incorrect use can cause damage to equipment and instruments and be harmful to staff members.

Activated acid or alkaline glutaraldehyde is expensive, unpleasant to handle if unbuffered, allergenic and potentially toxic. Treated equipment requires thorough rinsing. The efficacy declines after activation and with repeated use due to dilution and neutralising. If used regularly or continuously, a fresh solution must be prepared every day and kept in a sealed container. Reused solutions must be tested daily with special strips to ensure an active disinfection cycle. The manufacturer's instructions must be followed carefully, although these directions often do not take into account the type and frequency of use when determining expiry times. Therefore, if the quality of the solution is doubtful, it has to be tested or discarded. Exposure time of less than three hours is usually unacceptable for sterilisation, depending on the specific product used.

All workers regularly in contact with or responsible for chemical sterilisation must be informed of the risks to their health plus the uses and advantages/disadvantages of the method. Regular occupational health monitoring is indicated for all workers in contact with chemical substances.

Irradiation

This sterilisation method is used in industry to sterilise gloves, pre-packed disposable instruments, wound packs, clothing and foodstuffs.

6 | Clinical practice and procedures

Standard infection and prevention control precautions

With infection prevention and control, the risk and level of exposure to possible/probable pathogens dictates the measures needed to protect patients and healthcare workers. Since 1985, the Center for Disease Control and Prevention (CDC), Atlanta, USA, has promoted the strategy of standard blood and body fluid precautions in all healthcare settings, stressing that all patients should be assumed to be infectious for HIV and other blood-borne pathogens until proven otherwise. Standard precautions should be used in the care of all patients, including those in emergency care settings in which the risk of blood exposure is increased and the infection status of the patient is generally unknown. When emergency and public-safety workers encounter body fluids under uncontrolled, emergency circumstances in which the differentiation between fluid types is difficult, if not impossible, they should treat all body fluids as potentially hazardous.

Summary of standard precautions

- Avoid skin or mucous membrane contact with blood and body fluids. The skin or mucous membranes must be washed immediately if contamination occurs.
- Wash hands immediately after removing gloves.
- Wear protective clothing when the risk of significant, direct blood contact between the skin or mucous membrane exists, or is anticipated. This includes wearing gloves, masks, protective head- and eyewear, gowns or aprons.
- Dispose of sharps safely – do not remove a needle from a syringe, bend, break or otherwise manipulate needles by hand. Dispose of sharps in puncture-resistant containers kept at hand in the work area.
- Take care during injections, venepuncture and other vascular or minor invasive procedures.
- Deal with blood spillage correctly and immediately.
- Prevent injuries caused by needles, scalpels and other sharp instruments or devices.
- Avoid unprotected mouth-to-mouth resuscitation. Resuscitation bags, mouthpieces or other ventilation devices should be available.
- Refrain from direct patient care or handling patient-care equipment when suffering from weeping dermatitis or exudative lesions.
- Be especially familiar with and strictly adhere to precautions to minimise the risk of transmission of pathogens such as HIV or cytomegalovirus when pregnant.

Baby bottles, breast milk and feeds

Objective

Only pasteurised/sterile baby bottles and aseptic preparation techniques are utilised for preparing and handling breast milk and baby feeds.

Procedure

Handling used baby bottles

- **Maternity department and Nursery:** After each feed round, the used baby bottles (with tops and teats) and the warming jugs must be collected from the Nursery/Special Care Unit and sent to the receiving area of the milk kitchen.
- **Other paediatric departments:** After each feed round, the used baby bottles, tops and teats must be collected, rinsed in cold water and sealed in a clear plastic bag which can then be transported to the receiving area of the milk kitchen.

    The baby bottles must be rinsed with cold water and then washed with soap and water, using a dedicated bottle brush.

    The washed bottles must be disinfected (or sterilised), using one of the following procedures:
    - Steam sterilised in a dedicated preset autoclave for 20 minutes at 120°C, cooled, sealed with the cover and screw top and then packed in baskets or clean plastic bags.
    - Steamed upside down in a microwave oven with water in a special bottle container for the minimum period specified by the manufacturer (or at least 20–30 minutes) before packing and storage.
    - Filled with warm water, placed in a basin also filled with warm water and brought to the boil in the microwave oven for ten minutes (from when the water in the bottles starts to bubble). The bottles must then be left standing in the basin to cool a little before emptying each one, shaking it dry and sealing it with its cover and screw top. (Microwave ovens need fluids to heat a container and cannot be used directly on 'dry' bottles.)
    - Fill washed bottles with boiling water, place in a pot filled with water and heat on a stove or hotplate until the water bubbles for ten minutes (from when the water in the bottles starts to bubble). The bottles must then be left to stand in the pot to cool a little before emptying each one, shaking it dry and sealing it with its cover and screw top.

- The disinfected bottles can be held in the milk kitchen's clean store or sent to the paediatric departments for use.
- In smaller healthcare facilities or at home, the bottles can be packed and stored in the freezer compartment of the refrigerator, taking care to rotate the stock to ensure that the first bottles in are also used first.

Used teats

- The teats must be rinsed with cold water and rubbed with coarse salt before being washed with water and dishwashing soap.
- The rinsed teats must be boiled in water for 10 minutes (the boiling period starts when the water begins to boil) and left to cool in the pot with the hot water.

Handling clean bottles

- Staff who work in the milk kitchen must wear protective clothes (plastic aprons, masks, sterile gloves and paper caps).
- Hand-washing and disinfection between the different steps during formula preparation is of extreme importance.
- The milk must be prepared according to a recipe/directions and poured into the clean prepared bottles, identified with the baby's name, and placed in the refrigerator.
- No unauthorised persons may gain access to the clean bottles in a milk kitchen or storeroom.
- Filled, identified baby bottles must be transported to the patient care areas as quickly as possible and then kept at 4–8°C in the refrigerator until required.
- Unused bottles must be discarded and washed every 24 hours.

Clean teats

- In the Nursery, the clean teats must be placed in a dedicated, sealed bucket in a solution of hypchlorine that is changed daily (at least 250 ppm free chlorine). A special pair of plastic forceps to remove the teats from the bucket must be stored with the handle protruding from a container with hypochlorite solution which is changed every six hours to ensure that the chlorine does not evaporate too much to be effective.
- Clean and used teats must never be stored together.

Additional information

- Only sterile water/well-boiled water must be used in the formulas for baby feeds.
- The kettle in the milk kitchen must be decalcified regularly. If an urn is used, the tap must be disinfected at the same time the work surface is cleaned and disinfected, before mixing the formulas.
- The bottle brushes must be washed and boiled for three (3) minutes daily.
- Measuring cups, spoons, bowls and work surfaces must be washed with water and dishwashing soap and dried after every specific mixing procedure.
- Two sets of cleaning equipment (one each for the receiving area and the clean area of the milk kitchen) must be stored separately and kept dry between usages.
- The two areas must be cleaned separately – first the cleaner milk preparation (mixing) area and lastly the receiving area.
- Strict access control to the milk kitchen must be enforced when preparing the feeds.
- No unauthorised staff/person may gain access to the feeds. Feeds must be discarded if there is a possibility that they might have been contaminated/tampered with.
- The refrigerator must be washed out with warm water and detergent at least once a week, and when needed after spillage.

Breastfeeding and handling breast milk

Objective

Food, including mother's milk, must be handled with the highest level of aseptic technique to prevent the development of nosocomial infection, and prevent the wrong mother's milk being used for a baby.

Discussion

Though mother's own milk is normally not considered to be a great source of general infection, the milk can be contaminated and cause infection. The breast milk of mothers suffering from HIV/AIDS does contain virus, with varying concentrations, depending on the functioning of the mother's immune system. HIV-positive mothers must receive counselling before deciding whether to breastfeed or not. **Breast milk from HIV/ AIDS sufferers must NEVER be given to other babies.**

Other infections are more prevalent due to the contamination of expressed milk with micro-organisms.

Infection in breast milk may originate from:

- The mother's skin, which may not have been properly washed with soap and water before breastfeeding, or may have broken, infected nipples.
- A breast pump not properly cleaned or pasteurised.
- Parts of the breast pump that have remained soiled after improper washing, e.g. the pump was not disassembled beforehand and the rubber seal harboured contamination.
- Contaminated soap (especially communal bars or broken splinters of toilet soap that are used by everybody in bathrooms, cracked and soiled soap, or bars that lie in pools of dirty water on the rim of the wash basin).

- Contaminated and unwashed washcloths, also used to bathe the rest of the body and genitals.
- Adding freshly expressed milk to older, previously expressed milk to use as a bottle-feed. Expressed breast milk must not be stored for hours to be used again later. If milk has to be stored, it must be placed in a clean bottle in the refrigerator and kept at 4–8°C.

If the baby is bottle-fed with breast milk, the expressed mother's milk must be handled as aseptically as possible as it can be contaminated as easily as milk formula or cow's milk.

Staff must work with gloves when handling mother's milk. Following the principle that all human body fluids are considered infectious, breast milk has the potential of contaminating another person's hands/clothes or body.

Blood management

Objective

Staff must know and understand the procedures for safe blood handling and transfusion in order to minimise the risk of transmitting blood-borne infection. Diseases such as syphilis, malaria, infection with the human immunosuppressive virus (HIV) and hepatitis are blood-borne. A suspected 30% of South Africans are carriers of hepatitis B. Staff working with blood products should be aware of the implications of these facts.

Procedure for maintaining safety during blood transfusion

In principle a patient's body fluid and blood is always seen as infectious. Although blood for transfusions is assumed to be non-infectious, standard measures are utilised for handling all blood, irrespective of the source it comes from.
- Whoever has handled the transfusion bottle/

unit must wash their hands thoroughly afterwards.
- If there is a possibility that blood may splash during exchange of units or replacement of administering sets, the healthcare worker must wear protective gloves as well. Hands must be washed after removal of the gloves.
- Empty bottles/bags must be sealed in a transparent plastic bag and kept at 4–10°C in the refrigerator for 24–48 hours for cross-matching, should the recipient develop a transfusion reaction. These empty containers are a definite health risk due to blood leakage. After a container's holding time has passed, it must be discarded, still sealed in the plastic bag, in a sharps or medical waste container.

Procedure after exposure to blood and human body fluids

The following procedure is to be adhered to if a person has been in contact (splashes or splatter) with blood and human body fluids without using a barrier such as gloves:
- Wash the skin twice with hot water and antiseptic soap.
- Rub hands between the fingers and across the rest of the skin – friction removes at least 80% more micro-organisms than soap and water alone.
- Disinfect the hands with an alcohol-based disinfectant and allow it to spontaneously dry on the skin's surface.
- Report the incident to the supervisor if the skin is broken, to ensure that an injury-on-duty or incident-of-exposure report is completed.
- Complete an injury-on-duty report if the exposure is due to an accidental needle prick or other penetrating accident. (Refer to chapter 9, page 230).
- Rinse eyes after removal of contact lenses (if worn) with 0,9% sterile saline solution.

Cleaning spills of blood and human body fluids

The process for cleaning spills of blood and human body fluids is split into two steps or actions. Firstly, the spill must be cleared up and secondly, the contaminated area must be disinfected. The following points are important:

- The clearing-up must be done as soon as possible.
- Gloves are a basic essential, but plastic aprons and other protective clothing may be required if the contamination and the clean-up are extensive.
- The spill must be cleaned up with a paper towel, which must be disposed of into a medical waste container or colour-coded (e.g. red) plastic bag (destined for incineration).
- The surface must be washed with soap and water and dried with a paper towel. These must also be discarded into the medical waste container or red plastic bag.
- The area must then be then disinfected with paper towels soaked in a hypochlorite solution with at least 250 ppm free chlorine. The disinfectant must be mopped up to prevent someone from slipping or falling, if the spill is in an area such as a passage floor with a high traffic flow.
- A 1:10 solution of household bleach (one part fresh bleach in nine parts water) or a disinfectant releasing at least 1000 ppm free chlorine can be used on spills that may possibly contain HIV. A 5.25% solution of commercial sodium hypochlorite (fresh household bleach poured from the bottle) can be used in a 1:100 water solution.
- Remove gloves and dispose of them in the medical waste container or red plastic bag. Remove the container or bag for incineration.
- Wash hands.

Management of bloodstained equipment

Re-useable instruments and equipment

Bloodstained equipment must be rinsed with cold running water and sealed in a clear plastic bag. The contaminated items can then be transported safely to the appropriate reprocessing department where the staff can check through the contents of the bag, and then wash the items using gloves, detergent, lukewarm water and instrument brushes.

Disposable instruments

The worst of the blood must be rinsed off with cold running water before the item can be sealed in a sharps container, red plastic bag or medical waste box and placed with the medical waste for incineration.

Linen and pillows

Place these in plastic laundry bags and send to the laundry's sluicing facility. (Refer to page 150), OR rinse with cold running water and wash with detergent in warm water (at least 60°C) in the laundry. The physical removal of soiling through a combination of friction, detergent action and warm water lowers the biological load on surfaces and ensures that processes such as cleaning and pasteurisation are effective against the residual micro-organisms. Items must be tumble-dried and ironed if it is impossible to dry them in the sun.

Clothing

Place clothing in transparent plastic bags and hand it to the family for washing or send it to the laundry if there is a facility for private laundry items.

Non-washable items such as mattresses soiled with blood

If the items are not dry-cleanable, they must preferably be replaced. Items such as pillows and mattresses should always be covered with waterproof covers. Because some viruses such as hepatitis B can be resistant to heat, even a process such as steam autoclaving is not always going to make bloodstained bedding safe.

Bloodstained wound dressings and medical waste from patient-care areas

Seal the contaminated used item in colour–coded (e.g. red) plastic bags and place it with the refuse for incineration.

Please also refer to the discussion on waste management on page 152.

Bolus and tube feeds

Objective

Staff must know and be able to apply procedures surrounding bolus and tube feeding in a safe and competent manner, without risk of cross-infection. Safe procedures are necessary because hospitalised patients are more exposed and susceptible to infected food than healthy people in the community. Centralised food preparation increases the risk of infections as a single break in kitchen hygiene exposes a large number of people to infection. Where therapeutic liquid-bolus supplemental feeds and tube feeds are involved, the risk of infection is even higher because the technique of administering the feeds plays a role as well. Staff must be aware of the risks.

Procedure

Supplemental feeds usually consist of a single item such as a drink, a piece of fruit or some dry biscuits, given at regular intervals to patients who need supplemental feeds.
Tube feeds may also be given supplementally or be the total enteral nutrition of the patient. Tube feeds are given as:
- a bolus at regular intervals, administered with a syringe through a nasogastric or gastrostomy tube.
- a continuous infusion where the administering set is connected to a feed bottle that is regularly renewed.

Liquid-bolus supplemental feeds are usually given to a patient who cannot ingest enough calories or nutrition by eating. The additional drinks or snacks are meant to complement the main meals. Sometimes the patient skips the supplemental meal because he already has had a meal, is no longer hungry/thirsty or has a weak appetite. The items are left standing in the open at the patient's bedside. Micro-organisms that normally appear in very small numbers in any food or have been deposited in the food during preparation now start to grow without restraint, especially in sweet, dairy or protein mixtures containing milk. Even a small number of micro-organism (less than 10 000 cfo/ml) may form enough toxin to cause severe illness.

Bolus and tube feeds are not usually boiled or cooked during preparation, although boiled water may be used to reconstitute powdered ingredients. The feeds are usually slightly warm and must be cooled to less than 4–10°C as soon as possible, and stored in a refrigerator or other cool place. Uncooked fruit puree also turns sour very quickly if the fruit has not been boiled or washed well before preparation, even if it was peeled beforehand.

General

Feeding tubes must be irrigated with water:
- before and after administering medication
- before and after administering bolus tube feeds
- before starting and after ending an 18–24 hour continuous tube feed
- every four hours if bolus tube feeds are given.

Care must be taken to prevent aspiration – where possible, place the patient in semi-Fowler's position or lift the bed to a 45° angle during the procedure and for one hour afterwards.

Hints for safe bolus-supplemental feeds

- The food handler must wash his/her hands before and after the procedure. Contamination of the food is as great a risk as with tube feeds.
- Feeds must be stored in a refrigerator at 4–10°C. The amount of feed needed is measured into a clean, dry measuring jug in the kitchen or medicine room and the rest replaced in the refrigerator.
- All unused previous feeds must be removed and disposed of after each meal. It is false economy to store the feed for later use, as the quality of the ingredients will deteriorate.

Safe bolus tube feeds

Store feeds at 4–10°C in a refrigerator. The necessary amount of feed must be measured into a clean, dry measuring jug in the kitchen or medicine room and the rest replaced in the refrigerator.

In accordance with the hospital's policy, the position of the gastric tube must be confirmed and the presence of residual food in the stomach determined (e.g. by aspiration) before starting the next feed.

Liquid feeds are supposed to be administered with the assistance of gravity and must never be forced into the stomach. If the feed does not drain freely, 30 ml of lukewarm water can be carefully instilled into the tube and aspirated again to ensure that the tube is patent.

Prevent the syringe from emptying completely and air being introduced into the patient's stomach.

The tube must be carefully rinsed with 30 ml tap water and clamped. Make sure that both the patient's skin and the tube are clean and dry. Remove the used equipment, wash with dishwashing soap and water, store to dry or exchange at the sterilisation/pasteurisation department(s).

Unused tube feed that has stood at the patient's bedside for a time must be disposed of and never stored or reused or it will definitely give patients food poisoning.

Safe continuous tube feeds

The process is similar to that which has been described above, except that the feed bottle is connected to the gastric tube and the food is administered by gravity or with a feeding pump. No feed must hang for longer than 24 hours. The bottle with the residual feed and the administering set must be discarded as one unit when exchanged.

Hand-washing and hygiene

Objective

Staff perform procedures requiring aseptic techniques and surgically-clean patient-care procedures with clean hands.

Discussion

Hands should be washed:
- Before and after contact with the patient, his/her direct environment (i.e. the bed, locker), excretions, secretions, and all organic material such as blood, body fluids or tissue.
- Before and after the use of gloves.

Hand-washing is the single most important preventative/control measure against the spread of infection. Note the following points:
- Hands must be washed for at least 30–60 seconds with the appropriate soap, following

the correct procedure, with enough friction, and under running water.

- Special consideration should be given to washing the palms and the back of the hands, between the fingers, the sides of the hand and the finger tips, as these are the areas that usually receive least attention.
- Rubbing removes as many transient micro-organisms from the skin folds as soap and water, enabling the running water to rinse them away. If the water should splash over the basin and onto the clothes of the person washing, the environment becomes contaminated with the organisms from the hands. Cross-infection may follow.
- The first scrub for an aseptic technique such as a surgical operation must last at least one (1) minute to effectively clean the skin.
- Hands and other skin surfaces must be washed if contaminated items are handled or if hands are soiled with human blood, body fluid or tissue.
- Hands must be washed before gloves are donned and after they are removed, even if it appears as if the gloves are intact, as the skin perspires under the glove and more micro-organisms than normal are released from the hair follicles and skin pores.

Drying hands

- The use of a paper towel to dry washed hands is the most hygienic method available as the towel is used once and then discarded. Friction from the paper towel removes an additional layer of transient micro-organisms from the skin. Cotton or linen towels rapidly become a source of contamination as they harbour micro-organisms and allow them to multiply on the damp and soiled surface.
- Hot-air dryers circulate huge counts of micro-organisms that are sucked off the floor and then deposited on the washed hands. This drying process is also so time-consuming that most staff members do not wait for their hands to dry completely before rushing off. Cross-infection is thus encouraged. A dry environment is less hospitable to micro-organisms and they mostly die off more rapidly.

Hand disinfection/antiseptic hand rub

- Hand disinfection is always indicated before and after contact with the patient or his/her direct environment (i.e. bed and locker), even if there is no overt soiling of the hands with organic material or the patient's excretions/secretions.
- Hand disinfection before and after using unsterile gloves for a procedure is an additional protective measure.
- Disinfection before entering and after leaving the room of a patient in isolation (either direct or reversed isolation) ensures added protection for both staff members and patients.
- A mixture of alcohol and disinfectant with glycerin as emollient or a commercial hand rub product should be supplied in spray bottles that can be manipulated by the user's elbow. ± 3–10 ml of the solution can be sprayed into the palm of the hand and rubbed over the total surface of both hands until dry.
- Special attention should be paid to the fingertips, palms and sides, between the fingers and the backs of the hands. The process may be repeated between patient-care procedures/patient contact until the hands become sticky from the emollient. Washing with soap and water is then appropriate.

Additional information

- If bars of soap are used, they must be placed on a strainer that drains water and keeps the soap dry.
- If liquid soap in sachets or bags is used in wall-mounted dispensers, the empty bag must be discarded and not used for any other purpose.
- If the liquid soap dispensers have to be refilled, they must first be washed with a brush, then rinsed with warm water and left to drain/shaken dry before refilling. Just topping up is unacceptable.
- The use of sterile gloves for aseptic procedures does not replace hand-washing.
- Kitchen staff/food handlers' hands must be washed/disinfected every time they enter the kitchen.
- Cleaning staff's hands must be washed after they have completed a cleaning task. Working with soap and water does not automatically clean the hands.
- Dirty hands can contaminate clean cleaning solutions.
- Patients must be taught to wash their hands:
  - if they are visibly soiled
  - before and after meals
  - before medication is used
  - before and after procedures such as self-catherisation, or wound care
  - after soiled items such as bedpans have been handled
  - after coughing into the hand
  - after visiting the toilet
  - after contact with other people's skin, or with animals or birds.

Hydrotherapy (therapeutic patient bath)

Objective

Staff should know how to give hydrotherapy or a therapeutic patient bath that is both safe and beneficial to the patient. They should know that it is a procedure carried out following aseptic techniques for a patient who has a broken skin, multiple pressure sores or extensive wounds, such as burns, from which dressings have to be soaked loose.

Aims of a therapeutic bath

Hydrotherapy is a way to:
- loosen the patient's wound dressings without damaging the underlying tissue
- soften tissue before wound debridement
- apply medication to the skin or extensive wounds
- relax the patient's muscles so that passive movements or physiotherapy exercises may be done
- relieve muscle spasm or pain.

Procedure

This procedure requires at least two staff members to protect the patient against possible injury. The patient has to be bathed beforehand, as the body must be clean. The privacy/modesty of the adult patient or older child can be protected at all times by placing sterile towels over the private parts or allowing the patient to wear sterilised theatre pants if they are not in the way of the wound procedure. The following points should be noted:
- After each use, the bath must be thoroughly washed out with soap and water, rinsed and left to air dry. The outlet and fixtures submerged in the water, such as the plug, chain and shower head, must be washed as well, as human tissue often remains in the links or individual parts.
- Before hydrotherapy, the bath must be disinfected with a chlorine-based disinfectant and left for 10–20 minutes to disinfect all the fixtures. The outlet, plug, chain and shower-head must be disinfected. The disinfectant must be rinsed out with tap water before the bath is refilled, to prevent

irritating the patient's wounds/skin.

- The attending doctor must prescribe the bath on the treatment chart and specify what medicinal agent (such as 0.9% saline or 0.5% chlorhexidine, if any) is to be added to the water. The nursing staff should always check the prescription(s) before completing the treatment.
- The lukewarm water and additive must be mixed into the bath and again left for 10–20 minutes to disinfect the surfaces and fixtures.
- The temperature of the water must be checked to ensure that it is not too warm or cold, as a patient with burns cannot regulate his/her own body temperature and will very quickly become hypothermic. Normally a temperature of 35°–36°C (as for a baby) is recommended, taking the patient's comfort into account.

Wound care procedures

- Remove any loose dressings, without pulling or tearing the wound bed, and help the patient into the bath.
- Leave the patient to rest in the bath, with supervision, while the staff put on plastic aprons, (sterile) theatre gowns, (sterile) gloves, masks and caps. Remember – this is a wound care procedure, not a normal bath.
- Soak the rest of the dressings and only remove after they have loosened sufficiently.
- If the patient vomits or passes faeces in the water, the water has to be drained and the procedure repeated as the wounds have been contaminated and cannot be cleaned with soiled water. Because urine is usually sterile, urination in the bath is not a problem.
- Debride the wound (remove dead tissue) with sterile forceps and scissors or by gently rubbing the wound with sterile gauze.
- Clean and wash the wound surface by spraying it with the shower head and massaging the wound with the stream of water.

- **Test the water temperature first.** Ensure that the water will not chill or burn the patient.

Relaxation procedures

- The basic procedure is the same as for wound care, except that the patient is allowed to wear underwear or a swimming costume.
- Usually no disinfectant is added to the heated water.
- The patient can carry out any activity such as listening to music, reading, playing with bath toys, or blowing bubbles, but the staff must be attentive and ensure the patient's safety.
- Children younger than 10 years or mentally handicapped patients must never be allowed to bathe alone or be left unobserved within reach of a hot water tap.

Incineration of human tissue

Objective

Staff must understand and be able to apply the legal requirements for handling human tissue that is destined for incineration. They must know that human tissue must be handled in a specific manner because it is subject to prescribed procedures.

Definition

Human tissue destined for incineration usually consists of:

- tissue from operation theatres and delivery rooms
- tissue and specimens from the laboratories
- stillborn/aborted foetuses (pregnancy duration of maximum 26 weeks or a body mass of 1000 g or less).

Procedure to deal with amputated/ dissected tissue

NB! Find out what the patient's religion is before the anaesthesia/theatre consent forms are completed. Some religions, such as the Muslim religion, require that previously amputated limbs/ placentas/other body tissue be buried along with a deceased person and therefore the patient's family remove the tissue for safekeeping themselves. This MUST be noted on the theatre forms.

Weekdays

- The removed tissue must be sealed in a specimen container indicating that the contents are meant for incineration.
- The contents and patient's data must be written on a label and attached to the container.
- A lot-number must be assigned to the container in the theatre.
- The recovery room nurse must complete an incineration application form in duplicate and send the container and the copy of the documents to the incinerator.
- The original copy must be filed in the theatre incineration register.
- The delivery person signs for receipt of the container in theatre and takes it to the incinerator.
- The incinerator operator signs for receipt of the container and both the operator and the delivery person ensure that the container is incinerated.
- They sign the duplicate and a tissue incineration certificate is then issued with the date, the lot number of the container and the incinerator operator's signature on it.
- The duplicate request form must then be returned to the theatre and filed.
- The tissue incineration certificate must be filed in the patient's records.

After hours

The identified container of tissue must be placed in the mortuary/theatre refrigerator until the following working day when the incinerator is functional again. The 'weekdays' procedures can then be followed.

Foetuses

- Still-born babies with an intrauterine life of less than 26 weeks are not buried unless the parent(s) choose to do so, but are usually incinerated by the hospital where the delivery was done.
- Dead babies who have been delivered alive must be buried, even those younger than 26 weeks or weighing less than 1000g. The attending doctor must complete a death certificate in triplicate. The baby can then be handled like any other deceased patient in the hospital.
- If the parents insists on removing the remains for burial, the nurse in charge of the department must complete a special statement to that effect in triplicate, without using carbon paper, because three original copies are required. Both parents and the nurse must sign every copy of the statement (an original signature on all three) and all three copies must be verified by stamping with the hospital's official identification print. One copy must be placed on the mother's file, one handed to the parents, and one filed in the patient-care unit with the Request for Incineration forms. The identified foetus must then be placed in a plastic bag and handed to the parents.

Weekdays

- The foetus must be placed in a specimen container and identified with the mother's name.
- A lot number must be assigned to the container and documented in the labour room register.
- An official form requesting incineration of a foetus must be completed in duplicate and must be signed by both the parent(s)

and the attending doctor (without using carbon paper), and the copies stapled together.

- A staff member and a porter must take the foetus and the incineration forms to the incinerator, or else the hospital's delivery person must receive the container for transport after signing for its receipt in the labour ward.
- The incinerator operator must sign for receipt of the container on both copies of the form and both the operator and the delivery person must ensure that the container is incinerated.
- After incineration, a tissue incineration certificate is issued with the date, the lot number of the specific container and the incinerator operator's signature on it.
- Both copies of the form are returned to the labour ward, and the original is stapled into the mother's file, with the tissue incineration certificate. The copy of the original is filed in the labour ward's incineration register.

After hours

- The staff member must put the container in the refrigerator or freezer in the maternity ward.
- The foetus's data must be recorded in a special register.
- On the first working day when the incinerator is operational again, the procedure described above must be followed.

Placentas from the labour ward

- A rigid, leak-proof container with a sealable lid should be kept in the sluice room in the labour ward, or inside a special refrigerator/freezer dedicated to this purpose.
- Placentas must be placed in the container after examination.
- When the container is full, the lid must be sealed and the container sent for incineration.
- The labour room nurse must complete an incineration request form in duplicate and send the container plus one copy of the form

to the incinerator with a delivery person.

- The original copy must be filed in the labour room incineration register.
- The delivery person must sign for receipt of the container and take it to the incinerator.
- The incinerator operator then signs for receipt of the container. Both he and the delivery person must ensure that the container is incinerated.
- Both sign the duplicate form. A tissue incineration certificate can then be issued with the date, the lot number of the container and the incinerator operator's signature on it.
- The duplicate request form must then be returned to the labour room and filed in the incineration register.
- The tissue incineration certificate must be filed in the patient's records.

Embryonic tissue after an abortion outside a healthcare facility

It is usual for a woman who has aborted to take the aborted tissue back to the clinic or patient-care unit where the induction was performed to ensure that the placenta and other pregnancy products have all been passed. The tissue can then be disposed of in a container destined for incineration. The same process as for incineration of placentas should be followed.

Intravenous fluid therapy

Objective

Patients receive optimal care whilst receiving intravenous fluid therapy. Fluid therapy must be administered in such a manner that infections usually associated with the process are prevented.

Description

Cannula-related infections are usually endemic (coming from or involving a single patient), while drug-related infection (infection caused by a contaminated drug or intravenous fluid) may be the precursor of an epidemic. Cannula-related infections may present with or without fever and bacteraemia. (Refer to the discussion on page 121 for more details.)

Procedure

Hands must always be washed before and after any intravenous-related procedure, as well as before and after an administering set has been handled.

Strict aseptic technique must be utilised to start an infusion and to change infusion bottles/bags.

Introduction

The upper limbs are initially used to start an infusion. Only then are the lower limbs considered. The first site should be as distal as possible, with every following insertion wound more proximal than the previous one.

Skin preparation

- The skin should be cleaned with a swab soaked in povidone iodine, 70% isopropyl alcohol or chlorhexidine gluconate 0,5% in 70% alcohol.
- At least 30 seconds of swabbing in circular movements from the inside, where the proposed site of the entrance wound will be, to the outside is necessary.
- An area ±0,5 cm larger than the proposed dressing should be cleaned to prevent migration of viable skin micro-organisms from the surrounding skin to the wound under the dressing.
- The cleaned area must air-dry spontaneously and not be touched again.
- The cannula of an intravenous device must be well anchored to stop it from sliding in and out of the skin puncture wound, which contributes to the contamination of the device, vein and circulation.

- All the blood that has seeped from the wound must be mopped up with the alcohol swab before a transparent film dressing can be placed over the wound.
- Hair should be clipped with a pair of scissors before application, if adhesive plaster is used to anchor the device.
- Adhesive tape must never be placed over broken skin.

Peripheral intravenous cannula

- Peripheral intravenous cannulas should be replaced every 72 hours to prevent thrombophlebitis and infection developing, unless there is a shortage of usable veins or the puncture area is free of any sign of phlebitis or cellulitis.
- Insertion sites should be rotated.
- Lines set in position at a trauma or accident scene, or outside a hospital during an emergency situation must be replaced within 12 hours to prevent bacteraemia.

Insertion site (wound) care

- The area must be palpated carefully if sealed with a non-transparent dressing, and any pain, swelling or warmth documented and reported to the attending doctor.
- The appearance of the present insertion site must be inspected daily, as well as the appearance of other puncture wounds, so that any sign of inflammation and/or infection can be documented and reported as soon as possible.
- Wounds covered by transparent, semi-permeable dressings must be evaluated daily for redness, warmth, pain and sensation.
- Any complaints of pain or discomfort in the site must be investigated immediately.
- If the area is red, looks inflamed, or is swollen, the dressing must be removed immediately and the site visually inspected.
- The intravenous infusion must be discontinued and the cannula resited if any further redness, swelling, heat, pain or

drainage is observed.

- If the insertion wound drains pus or looks red and moist, a wound swab must be taken for laboratory microscopy, culture and sensitivity analysis.
- In the event that any thrombophlebitis, cellulitis or bacteraemia is suspected and/or confirmed, the infusion device, administering set and vaculiter must be removed as a whole.

Administering sets

- The rubber reservoirs of administering sets must never be squeezed, as this is one of the main ways in which blood clots, trace element crystals, or clusters of micro-organisms which are caught in the reservoir are forced into the blood stream.
- Each unit of intravenous fluid must only hang for a maximum of 24 hours before the container is replaced. Lipids and blood may usually only hang for a maximum 12 hours before replacement, while some of the newer hyperalimentation (total parenteral nutrition or TPN) solutions are stable and safe for a period of 24 hours. Check the specific fluid's guidelines.
- Administering sets must be replaced after 48–72 hours, as micro-organisms start to grow from the insertion site and migrate upwards at ±1 metre a day (biofilming). The set should be labelled with date and time of exchange.
- If filters or needle-less injection ports are added to the administration set, the manufacturer's guidelines should be followed as to how long the set may then be used. These devices guarantee greater safety, but are also more expensive to use.
- The administering sets for hyperalimentation must be changed every 24 hours.
- TPN containers often have their own dedicated administration sets that fit onto the container or a specific nutrition pump. Ensure that the correct device(s) are used

otherwise the transfusion may not work effectively.

- If blood, lipids or blood products have been administered, the sets must be changed before any other fluids are infused through it.
- The hub (connection) of the intravenous cannula must be disinfected with alcohol before a new administering set is connected to it.
- Used administering sets and empty plastic infusion bags must be disposed of in medical waste containers (e.g. red plastic bags) while sharp or blood-stained items must be discarded in a sharps container.
- After expiry of the holding time, blood-administering sets must be placed in medical waste containers for incineration.
- Opened administration sets must be handled as little as possible to avoid contamination. The open, unprotected end of the set must never lie directly on the patient's bed as this unavoidably leads to contamination/soiling.
- The inside of an unused administering set is sterile as long as the sheaths still cover the two open ends, while the outside is only clean and should not be placed on a sterile tray.

Central venous and tunnelled lines

- Central venous and tunnelled lines must be marked with the date and time a transparent film dressing was applied.
- Sterile gloves are required when the entrance wounds of central venous lines are handled.
- Luer-lock caps, lumen and needle-less injection ports must first be disinfected with a 70% alcohol swab before the caps are screwed or unscrewed.

Abba (additional/added-on) lines

- The smaller infusion bag must always hang higher than the bigger bag where a second infusion is coupled to an existing intra-venous line with a separate administration set or a Y-set as the added height (gravity) ensures a better flow.

- Again, the smaller bag/bottle must be hung as high as possible above the larger one if the infused fluid backs up into an empty smaller vaculiter on a closed line. Do NOT disconnect the smaller bag. The bag and set become contaminated during this process. Ensure that the intravenous device site or patient's arm has been immobilised and that the intravenous device is in the correct position in the vein.
- These administering sets are replaced when the main line is changed.
- A metal extension hook can be used to lower the main vaculiter below the level of the side vaculiter when both are in use and the smaller vaculiter does not flow well.

Handling additional added-on intravenous administration sets

- Handling empty added-on containers for patients receiving intravenous antibiotics or other medication through a second, sep-arate administration set often causes prob-lems. After an additional (small) vaculiter is empty, the flow regulator on the admin-istration set is closed and the vaculiter is **left connected** to the main infusion line. Staff members should be prevented from disconnecting the line and reinserting the contaminated needle into the vaculiter. A disconnected administration set that has been handled in such a manner **may never be used again** as the needle contaminates the remaining fluid in the vaculiter, which is usually left to hang for hours at room temperature. Pathogens start to multiply in the remaining fluid, migrate to the admin-istration set and are infused when a new vaculiter is connected. If the infusion set is left undisturbed, a new vaculiter may be

connected to it without having to replace the set and needle more than once in 24 hours, saving costs.

- If the main infusion flow is disturbed by the added-on line, the empty small vac-uliter must be elevated to enhance the effect of gravity on the infusion fluid in the main line or placed on an infusion pump.
- When the added-on set is replaced or removed, the needle is discarded into a sharps container and the empty vaculiter(s) placed in a waterproof medical waste container.
- Additional lines that are often connected and disconnected must be replaced every 12 hours as they are more often exposed to handling, air and environmental micro-organisms.

Antibiotics in side (additional) lines

Follow the procedure as discussed under added-on lines.

In critical care units, the lines have to be replaced often because there is sometimes a shortage of infusion pumps or connection sites on a multi-flow port. At times lines are physically removed so that a new administer-ing line with an additional vaculiter contain-ing a new additive can be started. There is a risk of contamination when this occurs. The different administration sets must be marked with the contents and disconnected from the main line with washed hands. A new, capped, sterile needle must be connected to the disin-fected, open end to keep it clean, and the whole placed in a clean plastic bag which can be stored on the patient's locker or in the refrigerator until needed again.

The new vaculiter must be connected to the administering set in use, the injection port disinfected with an alcohol swab before the new sterile needle is carefully inserted into the disinfected port/Luer-lock, the hub also disinfected and the administration set connected to it.

Additional measured infusion chambers: (or similar line extensions, most often used in paediatric departments) are managed as extensions of the administering set and medication is added in the form of bolus injections (described on page 186).

General

- If the healthcare worker's skin has been contaminated with blood during the procedure, the procedure must be completed as soon as possible and the skin washed with hot running water and soap, before disinfecting with an alcohol disinfectant. It is strongly recommended that the staff work with gloves when any venous puncturing procedure is being carried out.
- Used blood transfusion bags/sets must be stored in a transparent plastic bag in the refrigerator for 24 hours' holding time to ensure that cross-matching can be done later, should the patient have a reaction to the blood.
- Bags/bottles of infusion fluid and mixtures must be checked for clearness before connecting to the administration set. The patient's name and registration number, the date and time, and vaculiter contents must be marked on vaculiters containing medication or special mixtures such as hyperalimentation.
- Intravenous lines must never be irrigated with a syringe and sterile saline due to the danger of emboli being dislodged in the blood stream or of causing bacteraemia when bacterial biofilms from the cannula are deposited in the blood. To check whether the intravenous device is still in position in the vein, lower the vaculiter to below the level of the patient's arm and observe whether the blood flows back down into the administering set. If it does, the infusion is still viable. If it does not, the infusion should preferably be discontinued

and re-sited with the attending doctor's approval.
- Air filters will be needed when glass bottles are used or if a vaculiter tends to develop a vacuum. Ordinary injection needles must not be used under any circumstances, and especially not pushed through the top of the plastic vaculiter.
- The filtering end of the air filter must be positioned above the neck of the bottle to prevent leakage of the fluid.
- Stilettos, lancets and used sharp items/needles must be disposed of in a rigid sharps container.
- **Bolus injections** must be administered through the special injection port in the administration set and never through the distal rubber reservoir. The port must be disinfected with 70% alcohol beforehand. The bolus injection must be checked to ensure that it can be administered intravenously, and then injected slowly, taking time. Bolus intravenous injections definitely contribute to the development of intravenous infections and cause irritation of the veins, thrombophlebitis and tissue necrosis if the intravenous device slips into the vein too far.
- Blood specimens should never be drawn from intravenous lines as the infusion fluid may influence the laboratory results and the line may become blocked.

Dangerous practices

- 'Pumping' or squeezing the rubber reservoir of an intravenous line that is not flowing properly. This is extremely dangerous as emboli can be dislodged or bacteraemia caused.
- Injecting sterile fluid or aspirating fluids through an intravenous device with a syringe to unblock it.

Management of sharp instruments/objects ('sharps') and percutaneous (e.g. needle-prick) injuries

Definition

'Sharps' are sharp/potentially sharp items such as needles, scalpel blades, glass items, sharp metal, empty glass ampoules and vials, discarded test tubes, staples, lancets, caps from infusion sets and the metal parts of intra-venous infusion devices.

Percutaneous injuries include any penetra-tion, cuts or damage to the skin by sharp objects. Percutaneous injuries are common during:

- caregiving procedures
- the cleaning of instruments
- disposal of needles and other sharp objects
- the handling of instruments after complet-ing procedures.

Prevention of injuries

- Prevent percutaneous injuries by never walking around with uncovered, used sharps. An impermeable used sharps con-tainer should be taken to where the proce-dure is to be undertaken or the blood drawn. The **user** must discard the used sharps into the container her/himself.
- Used sharps should never be thrown into ordinary refuse containers or left where children or uninformed persons can be injured.
- Needles should never be removed from syringes except when a second substance is to be injected using the same needle. In this instance a container such as a kidney basin can be used to receive the first syringe before disposal.
- The cap of a used vacuum tube needle must never be replaced by hand – rather anchor it against a rigid surface while care-fully inserting the needle into the opening. The whole is lifted up so that the cap slides down the needle shaft. Now it can be unscrewed and safely discarded in the sharps container.
- **Four golden rules of needle-use:** Needles may never be:
  - recapped
  - bent or broken
  - removed from the used syringe, or
  - otherwise manipulated by hand.

Management of percutaneous injuries caused by used sharps

- The injured area must be washed with hot water and antiseptic soap. The injury must be rubbed or squeezed to encourage bleeding.
- The incident must be reported to the supervisor immediately.
- Blood specimens must be taken to define the risk of infection to the injured staff member.
- A single specimen of clotted blood must be taken from the injured staff member and the necessary laboratory tests such as analy-sis for hepatitis B (HBV) and human immunosuppressive virus (HIV) requested.
- If a patient with an unknown infection sta-tus is involved in the incident, permission must be obtained to draw a comparative blood specimen from him. Both specimens are sent to the nearest virology laboratory.
- If the source of contamination is unknown, or the informed patient refuses to give a blood sample, a single specimen must be taken from the injured staff member and sent to the laboratory.
- If the patient is not capable of giving informed consent (e.g. due to impaired consciousness), the doctor in charge of the case may give consent for a blood sample to be taken.
- If the patient is known to be HIV-positive, no blood need be drawn from him/her.

- Whatever the outcome, pre- and post-test HIV/AIDS counselling is imperative for the injured staff member.
- At the time of injury, the employee should immediately follow the employer's policy on work-related injuries. The incident and follow-up care should be documented in the employee's health record.
- In cases where the hepatitis B blood test is antibody-negative, immunisation against hepatitis B should be considered. (Refer to the information on percutaneous injury on page 186 for more detail.)
- It is not always necessary to take a blood specimen from the patient. Due to the possibility of false negative results in the HIV window period, many exposed staff prefer just to use antiretroviral prophylactic therapy in any case.

Respiration/oxygen therapy/ mechanical ventilation and equipment

Objective

For staff to know and be able to apply the correct method of disinfecting respiratory equipment. They should know that disinfection prevents the development and spread of equipment-related respiratory infection in a hospital. Bacterial contamination of respiratory equipment must be prevented or lowered to such a level that the risk of equipment-related infection is avoided or reduced as far as possible.

The **respiratory equipment** to which these guidelines have relevance includes:

1. Humidifiers (with or without loose heating elements).
2. Loose filters for circuits.
3. Mechanical ventilators (intermittent, continuous mandatory or assisted ventilation).
4. Wall-mounted high and low pressure vacuum bottles with tubing and catheters.
5. Nebulisers, such as 'Bubble-jet' or small inhalation nebulisers.
6. Disinfectant bottles.
7. Respiratory supply containers (beside the ventilators in intensive, critical-care and high-risk units).
8. Oxygen masks, tubing and connections.
9. Oxygen reservoirs for anaesthesia machines and ventilators.
10. Ventilator reservoirs (water baths).
11. Ventilator/respirator circuits, including tubing and circuits, the expiratory valve, medication and water nebulisers, and humidifiers.
12. 'Spiders' including bottles, tubing and masks.
13. Ruffle tubing.
14. Anaesthesia equipment for reuse, such as face masks, endotracheal tubes, laryngoscopes and airways.
15. Instruments used in a patient's nose in the Ear, Nose and Throat theatre.
16. PEED masks.

Oxygen humidifying

Oxygen is humidified to prevent drying the mucosa of the airways. Two methods, namely nebulising and humidifying, are used to saturate the oxygen with molecular water, preferably at body temperature.

Nebulising produces drops as well as molecular water suspended in the oxygen. Nebulising tends to cause more infections than humidifying as the drops are large and cold, and the fluid is easily contaminated. This leads to contaminated aerosols being released.

Humidifying produces molecules through heat or oxygen bubbling through water without large drops forming in the oxygen. Humidification may lead to contaminated aerosols.

Procedure

- Although steam autoclaving is the ideal way to process respiratory equipment, most of the items cannot withstand the high temperatures required. Sterilisation with ethylene oxide gas, disinfection with fluid chemicals or pasteurisation is indicated if the equipment is to be reused.
- All equipment must be disinfected before reuse:
  - Items 1, 3, 4, 5, 6, and 8–16 as listed above must be thoroughly washed with soap and water before pasteurisation.
  - Mechanical ventilators and machines (3) must be washed once a week and after each use, before disinfecting the outside with 70% isopropyl alcohol to ensure safety, especially if the machine has been used in another intensive care unit.
  - Suctioning tubing must be replaced daily and suction catheters wiped clean after each use and before disposal.
  - Disinfectant containers used to hold the end of the suctioning tubing must be emptied and rinsed before being sent for pasteurisation or sterilisation.
  - Respiratory supply containers must be emptied daily and washed with soap and water. To prevent contamination, only enough supplies per patient for the day should be placed in the container.
  - All equipment must be dry before storage.
- High-density air filters must be used in ventilator circuits to protect the patient from contaminated room air and/or gas, and to prevent retrograde contamination of the machine.
- Reusable ventilator circuits must be replaced every 24 hours (circuits without filters) or every 48 hours (circuits with filters).
- Only sterile saline or water should be nebulised. Unused pour bottles of water or saline should be kept closed and discarded within 24 hours after opening, as these fluids become contaminated very easily.
- Water baths and humidifiers must routinely be emptied, washed with disinfectant, rinsed and dried every 24–48 hours, as well as between patients, before refilling with sterile water just prior to use.
- Unused humidifiers and nebulisers must be emptied and dried before storage.
- Condensed water in ventilator circuits must never be poured back into the humidifier but be drained away into a separate container. Should this be done, contamination from the circuits would be transferred to the water bath.
- Multiple-dose medication vials for adding to humidifiers are easily contaminated. If possible, single-dose containers should be used and discarded. If multiple dose containers are used, they must be kept closed and dated at 4–10°C in the refrigerator for no longer than 24 hours before discarding.
- Equipment sets sent back to the pasteurisation or the Central Sterilisation Services Department (CSSD) must be complete and include all the parts so that these can be used again. If an item breaks, it must be marked and returned with the rest of the pieces and a report completed describing what happened.
- Only ever use clean, disinfected respiratory equipment.
- Disinfected and clean equipment not meant for immediate use must be reconnected/assembled and packed in a clear plastic bag to protect it from contamination.
- Water baths and reservoirs must be filled just before use and never be pre-filled and left for long periods.
- Heated water used in room humidifiers reduces the risk of transferring biological contagion from the water bath. Adding 25% acetic acid to nebulisers and humidifiers

prevents opportunistic pathogens such as pseudomonas from being released in the aqueous vapour. (Refer to the user instructions to check whether acid can be added to the water in a specific machine.)

- Routine random microbiological screening of processed equipment from the CSSD and the pasteurisation departments is a good indication that the system is functioning correctly.
- Mechanically heated washing processes such as found in circuit washing machines are quick, ideal and more reliable than chemical disinfection. If mechanical heating is beyond the means of a hospital, hand cleaning should be done as thoroughly as possible and heated processes used as much as possible.
- If chemical disinfection is done, the equipment must be rinsed off with sterile water (for sterile apparatus) or clean tap water (for unsterile equipment).
- Oral airway tubes and reuseable instruments used for procedures involving a patient's mouth or nose must be soaked in a solution of water and bicarbonate of soda before brushing with soap and warm water, followed by pasteurisation or chemical disinfection. All instruments must be surgically clean (aseptic).
- Equipment must be evaluated for cleanliness before use. If an item does not look clean or is defective, it should be exchanged and returned to the CSSD with an incident report.
- At the end of the theatre or clinic treatment list, the respiratory equipment should be disassembled, washed and appropriately disinfected/sterilised. Non-critical equipment such as nose-pieces of the oroscope can be pasteurised or soaked in a chemical disinfectant such as chlorine-based disinfectant or activated glutaraldehyde for 30 minutes.
- Reuseable vacuum bottles must be emptied

with care using gloves and a face mask, rinsed with cold water and sent for pasteurisation or washed with hot water and soap.
- If it is suspected or confirmed that a patient is suffering from pulmonary tuberculosis or any other contagious upper respiratory disease, all respiratory equipment such as circuits, masks, tubing and oral airways must be disconnected and washed with warm water and soap and the equipment sent for gas sterilisation.
- If an infectious disease is suspected during an operation, the gas compartment of the anaesthesia machine must be disassembled, washed with soap and water followed by disinfection with a chlorine-based disinfectant, before further disinfection/sterilisation according to the manufacturer's instructions.

Specimen collection for laboratory analysis

The main aim of culturing specimens collected from patients is the detection or confirmation of infection, as well as the identification and isolation of the causative pathogen(s). If requested, antibiograms are performed on the pathogens in order to determine which antimicrobials the micro-organisms are sensitive to. Microbiological surveillance allows the attending practitioner to identify the presence of infection and initiate treatment at an early stage.

Because both the diagnosis and treatment of the patient often depend on the laboratory findings, it is extremely important that specimens are always of a high quality, and should always be:

- Collected from the correct site using the appropriate aseptic technique at all times.
- Collected in the correct container (e.g. a catheter urine specimen may be collected in a sterile syringe capped by a sheathed, sterile needle).
- Collected so that there is a sufficient

volume/quantity to allow at least one or more tests to be done.

- Collected before antimicrobial agents are administered (e.g. before antibiotics are given intravenously or orally).
- Uncontaminated by skin cells, lint from bedding, soiled instruments or specimen containers.
- Labelled correctly with the patient's name, registration number and address. Specimens that contain suspected or confirmed contagious material (such as sputum for tuberculosis culture taken from a HIV-positive patient) should clearly be marked 'Biohazardous material'.
- Material meant for virus studies should be collected in the appropriate transport medium from the outset to prevent degeneration of the specimen.
- Taken from sites that were appropriately prepared before the procedure was performed (e.g. skin disinfection before venesection or lumbar puncturing).
- Collected with sterile instruments in sterile specimen containers with tight-fitting lids or caps to prevent contamination, leakage or spilling. The outside of the container should be uncontaminated to protect the specimen transporters and laboratory staff.
- Collected in the morning (generally), using the appropriate barriers (e.g. a face mask keeps drops of air exhaled by the healthcare worker out of the patient's specimen).

Transporting specimens

To prevent a loss of quality in specimens, it is important that they be transported to a laboratory as quickly as possible to prevent drying out or overgrowth with other quick-growing micro-organisms, such as normal bacteria, proteus or fungi. Some micro-organisms, such as anaerobic bacteria and gonococci, die so rapidly when exposed to air, that false-negative results may be reported.

They must also be transported at the correct temperature. Specimens that cannot reach a laboratory quickly should be refrigerated (4–10°C) **without freezing** as this causes cells to burst or dehydrate. Cooler bags and dry ice packs are ideal for keeping specimens cool.

Prerequisites for the request form

The patient's relevant clinical data must accompany the specimen to the laboratory via the request form. The information helps the medical microbiologist or technologist decide on the method of culturing and whether additional tests or alternative analysis in another laboratory are required. The balance between the clinical data and the laboratory results influences aspects of care such as the choice of antimicrobials, suggested surgery, continued hospitalisation or future treatment of the patient.

The request form must contain the following information:

- Identifying patient data (name, number, age, place of residence).
- Type of specimen (e.g. swab of granulation tissue).
- Date and time collected (corresponding with the date on the specimen, otherwise the laboratory might discard it).
- Clinical information:
  - date of admission
  - diagnosis/diverse diagnosis
  - occupational exposure, if any
  - history of illness (e.g. diabetes or renal failure)
  - date of commencement of the present complaint
  - previous/present systemic/topical antimicrobials that were/are used
  - type and anatomical collection area (e.g. aspiration of abdominal abscess)
  - analysis required (e.g. microscopy, culture and sensitivity analysis or MCS).

- Any known contaminants of the specimen (e.g. faeces on decubitus ulcers).

Specific specimen collection – suggested procedures

Only those types of specimens that are most regularly collected in healthcare facilities will be discussed.

Urine specimens

Clean catch (midstream) urine specimen

The success of these specimens depends on the patient's co-operation, understanding and technique, as collection is often explained and then left up to him/her. When improperly done, the specimen may be contaminated with material from the urethra; from the labia, vagina and surrounding skin of females or from the foreskin of uncircumcised males.

Suggested procedure if to be carried out by the patient:

- **Gather the following equipment before beginning:**
  - double-pocketed clear plastic specimen bag (or two attached plastic bags)
  - pair of latex gloves
  - refuse container with a plastic liner
  - solution of toilet soap and water in a basin
  - sterile kidney basin
  - sterile specimen container
  - antiseptic soap and paper towels
  - sterile swabs for washing
  - sterile water in a bottle.
- Ensure privacy by directing the patient to a toilet with a hand washbasin and a work surface on which all the equipment can be placed.
- Label the specimen container (this is done by the healthcare worker).
- Complete the request form and place in one pocket of the plastic specimen bag before starting the procedure, to prevent contamination of either. The healthcare

worker retains the bag.
- Explain the procedure to the patient.
- Wash hands and don the gloves.
  - **Female patients:** Hold the labia apart with one hand (the 'clean hand') whilst the other washes the vulva from the basin with the soapy water and the sterile swabs which are then discarded into the refuse container. The patient sits down on the open toilet and pours the sterile water from the bottle over the vulva – without letting go with the gloved 'clean hand'. Release the labia.
  - **Male patients:** Uncircumcised patients must carefully retract the foreskin without force as far as possible. Carefully wash the meatus with the soapy water and swabs. Pour the sterile water over the meatus into the toilet
- Pass some urine into the toilet to cleanse the urethral meatus of any contamination and residual soap
- Hold the sterile kidney basin by the rim and pass it through the stream of urine. At least 5–10 milliliters of urine must be collected and placed on the work surface.
- Male patients: return foreskin to position.
- (The patient may further empty the bladder into the toilet.)
- Pour the contents of the kidney basin into the urine specimen container. (Care should be taken to place the jar's lid upside down on the work surface to prevent contamination.)
- The container should be sealed before the patient rearranges his/her clothes.
- Remove the gloves, discard and wash hands.
- The supervising healthcare worker places the sealed specimen container in the other pocket of the transport bag before clearing up.
- WARNING: The patient should not void directly into the sterile specimen container unless it is wide enough to avoid contaminating the outside.

Suggested procedure if to be carried out by the healthcare worker:

The process is essentially the same except that the patient is placed on a bedpan and the practitioner washes his/her hands and wears gloves to complete the procedure. Patients who are unable to grasp the need for hygiene, who fail to understand the procedure, or are unable to use both hands will need assistance.

Urinary catheter specimen

Of all types of urine specimens, catheter specimens – especially those obtained from suprapubic catheters – are preferred by laboratories due to the lower level of contamination usually found.

Suggested procedure:
- **Gather the following equipment before beginning:**
  - double-pocketed clear plastic specimen bag
  - pair of latex gloves
  - sterile needle and syringe (10 milliliters)
  - alcohol or disinfectant swabs
  - antiseptic soap and paper towels.
- Label the specimen container.
- Complete the request form and place in one pocket of the plastic transport bag before doing the procedure, to prevent contamination of either.
- Explain the procedure to the patient, to ensure that he/she does not touch anything during the process.
- Clamp the catheter drainage tube below the specimen collection port and allow the tube to fill with fresh urine.
- Wash hands and don gloves.
- Disinfect the specimen collection port and allow to dry spontaneously.
- Collect at least 5–10 ml of urine with the sterile needle and syringe before recapping the needle **with the utmost care** to seal the syringe. Avoid contaminating the needle cap (sheath) whilst the specimen is being drawn.

- Place the capped syringe in the other pocket of the specimen bag so that the contents will not be ejected into the bag.
- Unclamp the catheter drainage tube and check the drainage.
- Remove the gloves, discard and wash hands after clearing up.

Sputum specimens

Sputum specimens are usually required to confirm or refute the presence of infection when respiratory pathology is suspected (or has been treated) in a patient. NB: sputum specimens should only be collected in well-ventilated areas, and preferably not in bathrooms or toilets where the ventilation is seldom good. This is done to ensure that the environment is not contaminated during the process.
- A sterile specimen container with a wide opening is required when sputum is collected by expectoration. Contamination of the outside should be avoided.
- The healthcare worker assisting the patient should wear gloves and a dustproof mask, especially if tuberculosis is suspected. Eye protection and a cap are necessary during endotracheal or nasotracheal suctioning, to prevent contamination of the specimen, the patient's airways and the practitioner's hair. Endotracheal specimens are usually more acceptable to the laboratory as they contain the least contamination.
- If the patient has poor mouth hygiene, gargling and rinsing the mouth with sterile water or saline will reduce the oropharyngeal contamination when the specimen is taken. Toothpaste or commercial mouthwashes will only decontaminate the mouth and oropharynx.
- Early-morning specimens are preferred, before the patient has brushed the teeth or eaten/drunk anything to contaminate the mouth.
- Only **coughed-up** material is acceptable.

If the patient **spits up** (without coughing), the specimen probably contains more saliva and not enough sputum or microorganisms. Only sputum will reveal the condition of the bronchi or lungs clearly.

Suggested procedure for collecting an expectorated sputum specimen:

- **Gather the following equipment before beginning:**
  - double-pocketed clear plastic specimen transport bag
  - sterile specimen container
  - antiseptic soap and paper towels
  - refuse container with plastic liner
  - paper tissues to wipe the mouth
  - sterile water in a glass (if necessary).
- Ensure privacy by providing a ventilated area with a hand washbasin and a work surface on which all the equipment can be placed.
- Label the specimen container.
- Complete the request form and place in one pocket of the plastic specimen bag before carrying out the procedure, to prevent contamination of either.
- Ensure that the patient washes his/her hands as he/she will handle the container.
- Explain the procedure to the patient and induce deep coughing. Children can be made to laugh, causing a coughing bout, but adults will actively need to cough. Vibration or percussion of the chest often helps.
- Hold the specimen container below the lower lip and ask the patient to carefully spit into it. At least 2–5 ml of sputum will be required.
- Seal the container and place in the other pocket of the specimen bag.
- Ask the patient to wipe his/her mouth with the paper tissue and discard it. Used and wet tissues should never be replaced in a pocket as they contaminate the clothing and hands of the user!

- Wash hands.
- Sputum should reach the laboratory as soon as possible. If it has to be stored for a while, refrigerate at ±4–10°C .
  (For collection of endotracheal aspirates, refer to page 203).

Stool specimens

Stool specimens can be used to identify pathogenic bacteria such as salmonella, shigella and campylobacter, or parasites that cause diarrhoea, such as giardia or amoebae, and protozoa such as *Trichomonas hominis*. The following points should be noted:

- A specimen jar with a wide opening is required. Contamination of the outside should be avoided.
- Stool specimens from infants can be collected by scraping the nappy for faecal matter.
- Stool that cannot reach the laboratory in time should be refrigerated at 4°C (in a separate refrigerator from the one containing medication or food).
- Healthcare workers collecting faecal specimen should wear gloves. Hand-washing is essential after they have been discarded.
- Rectal swabs are only taken if no stool can be obtained.

Suggested procedure:
- **Gather the following equipment before beginning:**
  - clean bedpan
  - clean spatula
  - double-pocketed clear plastic specimen bag
  - sterile specimen container
  - antiseptic soap and paper towels.
- Label the specimen container.
- Complete the request form and place in one pocket of the plastic specimen bag before carrying out the procedure to prevent contamination of either.

- Explain the procedure to the patient, provide the bedpan and ensure privacy.
- Collect 2–5 ml of stool with the spatula and place in the container.
- Seal the container and place in the other pocket of the specimen bag. The specimen should reach the laboratory as soon as possible.
- Remove and discard gloves and wash hands after everything has been cleared up.
- Microscopy for parasites: the specimen should reach the laboratory while warm. The parasites loose motility and die when the stool cools. If the cooled stool contains no cysts or eggs, the laboratory might not be able to confirm the results. If the specimen cannot reach the laboratory in time, it may be best if the patient is transported there. If the patient cannot travel, faeces can be kept warm in an ordinary vacuum flask especially reserved for stool specimens, following these guidelines:
  - Collect the specimen as described.
  - Pour warm water (37°C) into a clean vacuum flask with a wide opening (NOT boiling water, as this may cause the smaller container inside to burst).
  - Place the smaller container (with the stool specimen) inside the vacuum flask and the seal.
  - Transport the flask to the laboratory immediately.

Wound specimens

Wound specimens are usually taken during aseptic procedures and should be collected before the administration of systemic or topical antimicrobials and antiseptics. False-positive or negative results may be expected if the samples are taken afterward as they inhibit micro-organism growth. The following points should be noted:
- The use of gloves, masks, caps and plastic aprons is required for aseptic wound care procedures to prevent contamination of the patient's wound and the practitioner's face and body.
- Wounds are usually contaminated with micro-organisms and lint from dressings, endogenous micro-organisms (normal flora), transient foreign airborne objects such as dust and exudate.
- The seal of a sterile swab container should be checked before the sample is taken. Swabs with broken seals must be discarded immediately.
- Dry swabs are moistened in sterile saline solution or water to avoid rapid drying out and only non-viable micro-organisms reaching the laboratory.
- If the wound exudate is very fluid, the swab need not be pre-moistened.
- Tissue biopsy is more reliable than wound swabbing, especially for burn wounds or pressure sores. Deep tissue biopsies have to be collected under strict aseptic conditions – preferably in the operating theatre.
- Specimens may be refrigerated (at ±4°C) if transport to the laboratory is delayed.
- If a swab is taken from a sutured wound, one or more sutures may have to be removed to gain sufficient access. Re-suturing or closure of the open wound with adhesive strips may be required. Check with the doctor before sample collection.

Suggested procedure:
- **Gather the following equipment before beginning:**
  - double-pocketed clear plastic specimen bag
  - dressing pack and dressings
  - low-pressure vacuum with a sterile suction catheter and tubing (if necessary)
  - pair of sterile latex gloves
  - sterile wound swab
  - ampoule of lukewarm 0,9% sterile saline solution or sterile water (if necessary)

- sterile syringe with needle
- antiseptic soap and paper towels.

- Label the wound swab and disinfect the outside of the container.
- Complete the request form and place in one pocket of the plastic specimen bag before the procedure is done to prevent contamination of either.
- Explain the procedure to the positioned patient
- Remove the wound dressing, inspect and discard.
- Wash hands and don gloves correctly.
- Irrigate the wound with the sterile saline solution or water in the syringe to remove old exudate, contaminants from the dressings and exogenous micro-organisms.
- Gently retract the edges of deep wounds and irrigate the crater. The drainage fluid may be suctioned from the wound.
- Remove necrotic tissue to gain access to a clean wound bed .
- Gently rotate the moistened swab in a zigzag pattern over the wound surface, avoiding any remaining exudate, necrotic tissue, eschar and suppuration, as this only contains contamination and non-viable pathogens.
- Replace the swab in its disinfected container and seal.
- Complete the wound care. Antiseptic is only used on yellow (suppurating) or black wounds (the latter with the necrotic tissue incised so that the disinfectant may penetrate the wound crust). Red or pink wounds (non-suppurating epitheliasing) are irrigated with a sterile physiological solution of saline or water. Heavily exudating wounds can be 'washed' in a bathtub, using the shower head and clean chlorinated drinking water.
- Use sterile dressings to cover the cleansed wound.
- Remove and discard the gloves.
- The healthcare worker's hands are then washed, everything is cleared up and the patient is made comfortable.
- Place the specimen container in the other pocket of the specimen bag. The specimen should reach the laboratory as soon as possible.

Vascular catheter tips/portions of implanted devices for microbiological culturing

Indications for specimen collection

Skin site infection: Purulent drainage from the puncture wound accompanied by redness, warmth, pain, impaired movement, and positive culture. (A late sign of progressive infection.)

Pyrexia: Especially in patients with no other identifiable localised focus of infection and a central or other venous line in situ. Immune-compromised patients and the elderly may be infected without presenting with fever.

Phlebitis at the entry site of vascular or tunneled intravenous lines.

Positive blood cultures growing staphylococci or candida.

Colonisation of the insertion site or hub, confirmed by laboratory culture.

Hypotention: Consider septicaemia if no other clinical reason for continuous low blood pressure can be found.

Neglect: Open, unsealed ports left uncovered in a multi-port connection.

Classification of vascular catheter and implanted device infections:

Transient infection: Develops after any venous procedure such as venesection or intravenous injection.

Intermittent infection. After abscesses and localised infection such as pneumonia.

Constant infection. Due to conditions such as infectious endocarditis and septic thrombophlebitis.

Suggested procedure: **This is always an aseptic procedure.**

- **Gather the following equipment before beginning:**
  - sterile gloves
  - sterile equipment, e.g. a kidney basin, pair of scissors and forceps
  - two sterile specimen bottles marked to indicate which portion of the catheter/device they will contain
  - double-pocketed clear plastic specimen bag
  - face mask to protect the prepared wound area from respiratory contamination from the healthcare worker
  - plastic apron to protect the healthcare worker, and the wound area from potential contamination from the staff member's clothing.
- Complete the request form and place in one pocket of the plastic specimen bag before the procedure is done to prevent contamination of either.
- Wash hands using aseptic hand scrub with antiseptic soap and paper towels.
- Position the kidney bowl so that the distal (end) portion of the catheter can be placed in it.
- Clean the skin surface with a 70% isopropyl alcohol swab, using circular movements from around the catheter hub at the punc-ture site to the outside, cleaning a larger area than needed.
- Leave to dry for one minute.
- Remove the catheter/device and place it in the basin so that the hub hangs outside it to prevent contamination.
- Cut the bottom 3 cm (end) of the device off and place in the first specimen bottle with the sterile forceps.
- Cut a 3 cm portion of the catheter/device off just below the hub so that the part that was just below the patient's skin is included, and place in the second sterile specimen bottle.
- Clean the wound with a second alcohol swab and seal with an absorbent occlusive dressing.
- Remove the gloves, seal the bottles, dispose of the equipment and wash hands.
- Send the specimen to the laboratory immediately, with completed corresponding request forms.

Other/routine laboratory specimen

Routine laboratory specimen may be collected from the following sites: (Refer to table 6.1 on the following page).

Table 6.1: Routine laboratory specimens

ROUTINE LABORATORY SPECIMEN (to be taken by order of the attending doctor or the Infection Control Department)	TYPE
Blood specimen	Routine venesection
	Blood cultures
Cerebrospinal fluid (CSF)	
Faecal (stool) specimen	
Nasopharyngeal swab	
Penile swabs	
Skin scrapings	
Sputum specimen	Aseptic endotrachial aspirates (e.g. with a 'Luki' tube)
	Expectorated sputum specimen
	Sterile bronchial lavage (in theatre)
Throat swabs	
Urine	Urinary catheter specimen
	Clean catch/midstream specimen
Vaginal swabs	
Wound swabs	Infected wounds
	Routine monitoring of burns/wounds
Biologically hazardous specimen	
Suspected or proven viral haemorrhagic fever specimen, e.g. Crimean-Congo fever	All blood and body fluids
Suspected or proven viral infection specimen, e.g. Hepatitis A, B, C, HIV	Blood and body fluids
	Stool specimen
Environmental sampling	
Air	Centrifugal air sampler (theatre)
	Settle plates (theatre)
Hot water sampling	In cases of legionella infection in an institution
Surface sampling	Rodac plates (kitchens and laboratories)
Water	
Food sampling	
Infant's formula	
Food	After an outbreak of 4 or more cases of diarrhoea after a meal
Routine sampling of personnel	
Nasopharyngeal swabs	MRSA or MRSE outbreak

Table 6.2: Frequency of specimen collections

Patient sampling	Frequency
Suspected infectious patients Patients with diagnosed contagious diseases Patients with diagnosed transmissable diseases	When signs and symptoms of infection are observed, e.g. increased secretions, offensive smells, pyrexia, colour changes in wounds: ■ The doctor may order collection of specific specimens in the theatre ■ The infection control consultant may order collection of an appropriate specimen to monitor an outbreak of infection/the condition of a specific patient ■ The ward staff may collect the appropriate specimen in conjunction with the attending doctor
Private patients of specified physicians	As requested/ordered by the doctor
Patients with specific conditions (such as burns, bone marrow transplant)	Following a routine monitoring schedule or protocol

The laboratory results (microscopy, culture and sensitivity analysis or MCS)

- Macroscopic and microscopic analysis usually takes between 24–48 hours, depending on the amount of microbiological growth and the different types of micro-organisms in the specimen. A portion of the specimen is placed on a glass slide, stained and evaluated microscopically.
- Gram-positive and negative micro-organisms, leucocytes and epithelium can be seen and usually identified immediately.
- The rest of the specimen is transferred to a culture medium and incubated to induce growth.
- Immediate microscopy may give an initial indication of (possible) causative pathogens, allowing speedy treatment with a generally appropriate antibiotic in cases of life threatening infection.
- Culturing and the determination of antibiograms to assess the sensitivity of the pure pathogen to indicated antimicrobials would confirm or refute the initial choice of antibiotic.
- Completion of this final stage of determining sensitivity may require 2–5 days. In the interim, preventative and control measures should be applied against the worsening or spread of infection.
- Nursing staff must be taught to interpret laboratory results, especially in rural clinics and healthcare facilities that have no full-time medical doctor in residence. Knowledge of the results is necessary in order for healthcare workers to choose and initiate the appropriate infection control measures and chemotherapy.

Stoma care

Objective

Stomas are cared for in hospital using an aseptic technique so that patients do not develop incident-related nosocomial infection. A fresh stoma is an open, draining wound and aseptic technique is indicated, as the tissue initially is very susceptible to infection, including colostomies that excrete stool.

Definition of a stoma

There are three types of stomas:

1 A surgically manufactured temporary or permanent opening in a hollow organ that exits on the surface of the body, with the aim of excreting body waste (for example a colostomy, ileostomy, urostomy, cystostomy) or allows access to the lung (such as a tracheostomy).

2 A surgically manufactured artificial opening (mouth) into the stomach (gastrostomy) or jejunum (jejunostomy) through which the patient is fed.

3 A surgically manufactured temporary or permanent internal opening (anastomosis) that connects two hollow body structures, for example a gastroenterostomy, pancreatoduodenostomy or pyelo-utererostomy.

Procedure

Ensure that the patient is informed of what to expect prior to the procedure and is prepared for the appearance of the stoma and the fact that he/she will be need to be taught how to care for it. Remember that:

- The appearance of the stoma must be evaluated every six hours. A viable stoma is pink or red in colour, secretes mucus that does not contain yellow (possibly pus) or dark red (possibly bleeding) clots.
- The smell of the stoma must be evaluated as well – an offensive smell (not the smell of stool) with heightened drainage must be documented and reported to the doctor immediately. A wound swab of this stoma must be sent to the medical microbiology laboratory to exclude infection.

Excretory stomas

- In hospital all observations and procedures must be charted in the patient's records.

Any abnormalities must be noted and the patient's vital signs (temperature, pulse and blood pressure) monitored twice daily in order to identify the first signs of infection.

- Splints (tubes) in an **urostomy** must be handled with the utmost care as they keep the anastomosis open and create an excellent entrance for micro-organisms into the internal wound site. The tubes drain urine and must be sealed inside a stoma bag. A wound swab of the stoma must be sent to the medical microbiology laboratory to exclude infection if this wound starts developing an offensive smell.

- With a **cystostomy** the urine drains through an implanted suprapubic catheter into a collection bag or leg bag, which must be emptied every few hours. The skin fistula is cared for like other stomas and cystostomies tend to develop the same type of problems as urostomies. The same solutions work for both these problems.

- The stomal patient must be given a neutral diet to start with. Roughage is not promoted in the initial diet, as the intestine is tender after the surgery and the anastomosis must rest. Ileus or obstruction may also be a problem that can lead to gangrene.

- The person who will manage the stoma must wash their hands carefully. If the carer is a hospital staff member he/she must use gloves and a protective plastic apron. If the carer is the patient or constantly the same person at home, gloves are not necessary but hand-washing remains very important.

- If the stoma bag has two parts and the ring or cover plate which adheres to the skin is still usable, the skin and wound can be cared for inside the ring or plate without damaging the seal. The cover plate (without a ring) can only protect the stoma against external damage if the opening is the right size.

- During removal, the used stoma bag must be folded double so that one side sticks to the other. The bag must be discarded into a medical waste container or plastic bag. At home the used bag must be wrapped in newspaper and placed in the refuse.

- The patient's stoma is cared for aseptically. Hyperproduction of mucus must be removed with a piece of gauze and the area evaluated for signs of infection.

- The skin surrounding the stoma must be evaluated for redness and erosion. The area must be carefully washed either with sterile saline solution, dabbed dry with sterile gauze (if the procedure is done in hospital), or with mild toilet soap and warm water, and dabbed dry with toilet paper (if done at home).

- In urostomies, which excrete urine continuously, a sterile gauze dressing should be placed over the stoma itself while the peristomal skin is cared for.

- Colostomy stool can be either fluid, semi-fluid and corrosive or non-corrosive, or solid/formed and non-corrosive, depending on where the colostomy is sited. Colostomies of the right side of the colon and the transverse colon secrete a corrosive stool that may damage the patient's skin, giving rise to a secondary infection. The alkaline fluid stool excreted by ileostomies is corrosive and can cause erosion of the skin areas. Ileostomy patients must place an ordinary cover plate under the stoma bag or use stoma paste around the opening of the bag to seal it tighter.

- A bag with the correct-size opening and of the correct type must be placed over the stoma or clicked onto the ring/cover plate and carefully but firmly pressed down while the patient holds in his/her breath (without pushing out the stomach).

- The bag must be observed regularly so that it can be emptied when full, before the seal between the skin and cover plate breaks.

- Urostomies should be connected to a bag and allowed to drain freely at night so that

the patient can sleep.

- The patient must be taught how to manage the stoma bag and/or urostomy leg collection bag at home to ensure that the bag drains freely and no retrograde flowback to the stoma takes place. The patient must be given an opportunity to walk around and practise with the bag(s) while in the hospital.

- Urostomy patients must be taught to identify the signs and symptoms of urinary tract infection to prevent corrosion of the stoma.

- The colostomy patient must regularly evaluate the stoma for stricture formation so that the skin will not split should huge volumes of stool be passed.

- Skin infection is a problem for all stomal patients.

- Stomal aids are available to prevent damage to stomas and peristomal skin, e.g. cover pieces used as skin protectors to prevent tearing of the skin layers, skin preparation and cleansing agents, solvents that soften dried adhesive layers, special paste that seals bags closer, barrier creams and special pastes that will fill up tissue hollows and skin folds so that the bag seals better.

- Disposable stoma bags must never be washed out or disinfected and reused.

- Reuseable stoma bags, collection bags and leg bags are rinsed in cold water and filled with a vinegar-and-water solution for 30 minutes (0,5 ml vinegar in 750 ml lukewarm water). The vinegar solution helps to neutralise smells and the development of pseudomonas infection but the solution must be carefully rinsed out of the bag with cold water before reuse.

Feeding stomas

- A special feeding tube or catheter must be passed into the stoma and anchored with a suture or adhesive plaster until the fistula has formed (±2–3 weeks).

- The tube remains clamped until the patient is fed/hydrated/medicated.
- The tube must be rinsed through with ±30 ml clean water after the feed or installation has been administered, to avoid the remainder of the administration turning sour or to stop micro-organisms multiplying in the tube.
- Leakage of gastric acid and digestive enzymes past the tube can cause skin irritation or erosion.
- Encrusted tubes can be irrigated weekly with 30 ml soda water or other carbonated fluid.

Aseptic change of a feeding tube in a newly formed permanent gastrostomy

- Check the attending doctor's prescription to change the tube, or if the tube is blocked, check with a nursing supervisor who knows the patient.
- The caregiver must wash their hands and put on gloves, a plastic apron, mask and cap.
- Remove the old dressing and clean the stoma aseptically with sterile saline and sterile gauze. If the fistula has completely granulated, the skin may be washed with mild toilet soap and lukewarm tap water.
- Completely deflate the anchoring balloon with a syringe and remove the tube by pulling gently on it with a rotational movement.
- Lubricate the bottom 8 cm of the new tube with a sterile waterbased lubricant.
- Carefully pass the new tube through the fistula opening, using a rotational movement. If resistance is encountered, the tube must be removed and passed at another angle, e.g. inward or downward. The attending doctor must be contacted if the tube cannot be inserted at all.
- Clean the area around the tube gently with sterile gauze and replace the wound dressing before making the patient comfortable.
- Discard the used tube in a medical waste

container or (red) plastic bag.
- The gastrostomy aspirations and feeds must be administered as taught (similarly to a bolus nasogastric tube feed).
- No gastrostomy feeds should be administered if the patient is already nauseous or vomiting. The nausea should be reported and the attending doctor contacted if the symptoms persist beyond one feed/treatment period.

Suctioning the patient's airways

Objective

The objective of this procedure is to ensure that the patient has a patent airway. Infection prevention and control measures must be strictly adhered to at all times. Staff must know that suctioning a patient's airways is an aseptic and potentially contaminating procedure. Endotracheal suctioning especially carries a high risk of contamination of the patient, staff and environment. (Refer to page 193 and the discussion of the collection of a sputum specimen for more information). Staff must know the procedures to eliminate/reduce these risks.

Procedure

- All requirements must be collected beforehand so that the procedure may be completed without interruption.
- A new sterile suctioning catheter must be used for each procedure and discarded afterwards unless the patient has been fitted with a closed-circuit suctioning catheter (a catheter that has its own permanent protective sheath through which suctioning can be done for a period of 24 hours at a time).
- Suctioning equipment must be available at the bedside of mechanically ventilated patients or those with tracheostomies, as emergency suctioning may be urgently needed at any time.

- Eye protection, a mask and a cap are necessary during open endotracheal or nasotracheal suctioning to prevent contamination of the specimen, the patient's airways, and the staff member's face and hair.
- **Endotracheal aspirate specimens** are preferred by the laboratory as they contain the least contamination, especially if taken with a closed suctioning catheter.
- If a tracheostomy patient has poor mouth hygiene, gargling and rinsing the mouth with sterile water or saline will reduce the oropharyngeal contamination before the endotracheal aspiration specimen is taken. Toothpaste and mouthwashes only contaminate the mouth and oropharynx, and may actively suppress micro-organism retrieval.
- The conscious patient must be informed of the procedure, what to expect and how to co-operate.
- If possible, the patient must cough up as much of the secretions as possible before the procedure to try and shorten the suctioning period. By teaching the nursing staff how to administer chest percussion and stimulate the cough reflex, a physiotherapist can help a patient who cannot cough by himself.
- To make secretions more fluid, 2–5 ml sterile saline is installed in the endotracheal tube with a sterile syringe and left for one to two inspirations.
- The patient's head is carefully turned to the right to facilitate suctioning of the left bronchus.
- **Endotracheal suctioning should never be continued for longer than the average staff member can hold his/her own breath (± 15–30 seconds).** The patient must be given time between suctioning episodes to draw a breath or to be ventilated with oxygen for a few minutes (no less than 30–45 seconds) to prevent hypoxia and arrhythmia.

- Before suctioning commences the suctioning catheter must be passed through the endotracheal tube for 20–30 cm with a rotational movement (unless otherwise ordered or if resistance is encountered).
- The catheter must be removed if the patient coughs.
- Suctioning must be done using rotational movements, without dragging the catheter across the mucous. Contact with the side of the tube must be prevented to avoid contamination of the catheter.
- Reusable suction bottles must be emptied every six hours by staff wearing gloves. The bottles must be covered with a bedpan cover to prevent contaminating aerosols forming as the fluid in the bottle laps or is shaken. The bottles are rinsed with cold tap water and sent for pasteurisation every second day.
- Single-use disposable suction containers can be sealed and disposed of in a medical waste container or (red) plastic bag without emptying.
- The inner cannula of the tracheotomy tube must be replaced with a pasteurised/sterile cannula, or may be soaked in a solution of bicarbonate of soda and cold water to loosen all mucus, and washed with soap and a brush before rinsing and pasteurising in warm water at 65°C for 5 minutes. The outer tube must be suctioned clean before replacing the inner cannula.
- The procedure, as well as the colour, consistency, volume and character of the secretions, must be noted in the patient's chart.

Suctioning with an *open* catheter

- Small screw-capped bottles of sterile water can be ordered from the CSSD department to flush the catheters during open suctioning procedures. Each bottle must only be used for one procedure and the remaining contents discarded afterwards.
- Bedside bottles containing a disinfectant

solution for storing the end of the open catheter suctioning tube when not in use must be rinsed daily, before washing, rinsing, shaking dry and refilling with 100 ml of fresh disinfectant.

- The staff must wear sterile gloves, caps and aprons as protection against splatter and splashing drops and surgical masks to prevent the mutual exchange of aerosol-laden expirated air currents during aseptic endotracheal suctioning.
- Nasal or oral suctioning may only require the use of gloves, but endotracheal suctioning does justify the use of all the measures.

- A closed-circuit suctioning catheter must never be disconnected and left to lie on the patient's sheets, as the end becomes contaminated. Rather use a second vacuum tube connected to a catheter when suctioning the patient's mouth, and disconnect the tube at the vacuum **container**. The distal end of whichever tube is unused can be temporarily stored in a bottle of disinfectant to keep it clean until needed again. This means that there are always two suction tubes per vacuum device available at each bedside when closed-circuit suctioning catheters are used.

7 | Special patient categories

Admitting patients with suspected or confirmed infectious conditions

Objective

Staff, patients and the environment are protected as far as possible from infectious conditions.

On admittance to the healthcare setting, a patient's clinical condition is assessed, the medical history is taken and the complaints evaluated in order to make a preliminary nursing diagnosis. If the attending doctor prescribes it or the registered nurse feels that the patient's condition justifies it, the patient may be placed in a general ward or a private room with/without an en-suite bathroom. The following patients should preferably be placed in private rooms:

- patients with infectious airborne conditions
- the patient who cannot achieve or maintain a satisfactory level of personal hygiene
- susceptible patients with a low level of resistance to infection or serious immunosuppression that justifies placement in protective isolation, e.g. <200 white cells/ml blood
- terminally ill or dying patients
- patients with extensive open wounds exuding large volumes of body fluids or extensive second/third degree burns
- patients with multi-drug-resistant hospital acquired infection.

Mobile, incontinent patients with enteric transmissible conditions such as hepatitis, typhoid, cholera or any type of diarrhoea are admitted to rooms with en-suite bathrooms or placed near to a bathroom. Specific measures must be taken to keep communal facilities clean or to wash bedpans and urinals so that the safety of other patients and staff against contamination/soiling is ensured.

Universal (standard) preventive and control measures must be utilised to protect the staff, other patients and the environment against contamination/soiling. (Refer to page 171 for a discussion of standard precautions).

Dealing with death

Outcome

Supportive and efficient patient care is delivered to all patients during the dying period and after death, as in life.

Objective

When an infectious patient dies, the suspected/confirmed cause of death must be determined. The necessary measures to protect the staff, patients and the environment against contamination/contagion must be chosen accordingly. As all human blood, tissue and body fluid may remain infectious for days after death, protective measures are indicated when working with patients who have died. Material that was contagious during life remains so after death.

The nursing staff must make sure that any special measures are adhered to by the pathologist in cases where a post-mortem is to be performed on the patient's remains (e.g. that prosthesis or devices such as mechanical pacemakers remain in place).

There are some definitive rules in cases where an infected/infectious patient has died, which are detailed in the table below. After the patients' family has viewed the remains, protective measures must be utilised to protect all healthcare workers who have contact with the patient.

WARNING: These measures are only applicable to patients who are laid out by hospital staff. In some cases, only a religious personage, such as a Jewish Rabbi or other official is permitted to handle the remains – that person must then be warned of the possibility of infection, or its definite presence. This is applicable to the undertaker/funeral services as well.

Table 7.1: Suggested precautionary measures

CLINICAL OBSERVATION	INFECTION CONTROL MEASURE
Leakage of human blood and body fluid from the skin or any orifice	<ul><li>Plastic aprons</li><li>Hand disinfectant/hand-washing</li><li>Gloves (double gloves in cases of haemorrhagic fever)</li><li>Single or double plastic body bags</li><li>Seal all body openings with a layer of plastic or waterproof plaster. Place cotton swabs in the mouth and throat of the patient</li><li>Identify the outside of the bags with biohazard stickers</li><li>Write the biographic data of the patient on the outside of the bag</li><li>Contaminated linen: seal in colour-coded (e.g. yellow) plastic bags and transport to the sluicing facility or the laundry. Mark bags with biohazard stickers</li><li>Wash and terminally disinfect the bed and environment</li><li>Reuseable equipment/supplies: seal in colour-coded plastic bags (e.g. clear) for reprocessing. Mark with biohazard stickers if necessary</li><li>Medical waste: Seal in colour-coded plastic bags (e.g. red), pack in boxes, mark with biohazard stickers and send for incineration</li></ul>
Patients suffering from an airborne infectious condition	<ul><li>Plastic aprons</li><li>Masks</li><li>Hand disinfectant/hand-washing</li><li>Gloves</li><li>Seal all openings in the body as discussed above</li><li>Contaminated linen: seal in colour-coded (e.g. yellow) plastic bags and transport to the sluicing facility or the laundry, mark with biohazard stickers if necessary, e.g. varicella</li><li>Wash and terminally disinfect the bed and environment</li><li>Re-useable equipment/supplies: seal in colour-coded plastic bags (e.g. clear), mark with biohazard stickers and send for reprocessing</li><li>Medical waste: seal in colour-coded plastic bags (e.g. red), pack in containers, mark with biohazard stickers if necessary, and send for incineration</li></ul>

CLINICAL OBSERVATION	INFECTION CONTROL MEASURE
Patient suffered from a contact-transmissible infectious condition	<ul><li>Plastic aprons</li><li>Hand disinfectant/hand-washing</li><li>Gloves (double in the presence of extensive bleeding)</li><li>Seal all openings in the body as discussed</li><li>Contaminated linen: seal in colour-coded (e.g. yellow) plastic bags and transport to the sluicing facility or the laundry. Mark with biohazard stickers</li><li>Wash and terminally disinfect the bed and environment</li><li>Reuseable equipment/supplies: seal in colour-coded plastic bags (e.g. clear), mark with biohazard stickers and send for reprocessing</li><li>Medical waste: seal in colour-coded plastic bags (e.g. red), pack in boxes, mark with biohazard stickers, and send for incineration</li></ul>

Using plastic/waterproof body bags

Single bags

These are indicated for:

- All patients whose skin is not intact and have wounds/lesions that cannot effectively be sealed with a waterproof plastic dressing, e.g. where there are extensive abrasions or burns.
- All patients where there is a possibility of leakage of human blood and body fluid from orifices/openings in the body that can contaminate the healthcare workers, e.g. after a drowning, if the patient had a blood clotting defect or abdominal obstruction.
- Cases where the diagnosis is still unknown but the patient presented with fever of unknown origin and infection is suspected.
- Patients with suspected/confirmed infections such as HIV or acute hepatitis B.
- Patients who died from organophosphate poisoning.
- Patients with suspected/confirmed highly formidable diseases such as rabies and meningococcal meningitis.

Double bags

These are indicated for patients where extensive leakage of human blood and body fluid from the orifices/openings in the body or the mucosa/skin are a definite danger to the healthcare workers, e.g. where the patient has extensive uncontrollable interstitial bleeding ('DIC'), typhoid or a haemorrhagic fever such as Crimean-Congo fever.

Immunosuppression: protective/reversed patient isolation

Outcome

Patients in protective/reversed isolation receive high-level care under all circumstances.

Objective

Immunosuppressed patients must be housed and cared for in such a manner that the risk of infection is minimal.

Patients with a white cell count of 200 cells/ml or less are classified as immunosuppressed and should be placed in protective isolation. This includes patients with a low protective antibody count who have not been immunised, HIV-positive patients, patients suffering from malnutrition or metabolic abnormalities, persons on cortico-steroid treatment, organ or bone marrow transplant patients, as well as oncology patients on chemo- or irradiation therapy.

Procedure

- The attending doctor decides what the patient's immune status is, e.g. through assessing the white cell count and clinical condition.
- The patient and family are informed about the immunosuppression and what the procedure for protective isolation entails, to ensure their co-operation.
- Special protective measures against infection, such as strict barrier nursing and restricted access for a period of days to weeks, are often applied in bone marrow transplantation and chemotherapy.
- Although the patient must be treated as normally and routinely as possible for the sake of mental health, certain aspects of isolation are accentuated, which are detailed below.

Hand hygiene

As for direct isolation. Hand-washing and disinfection is the single most important measure to prevent cross-infection. The patient and family have to be taught to wash their hands before and after contact with the patient and his/her direct environment.

Single room

If possible, the patient is housed in a single room with an en-suite bathroom to prevent the spread of infection from a commonly used environment to the patient. The door should be kept closed to contain airflow from the rest of the ward. Due to the fact that these patients often develop claustrophobia and feelings of alienation, keeping the door open a crack might be necessary.

Protective clothing for the staff

The patient must be protected from contamination from the clothing of staff who have cared for other patients. The use of gloves is unnecessary unless an aseptic procedure is to be done or blood taken, or if the staff member may be contaminated with blood and human body fluids during a care procedure. Face masks (surgical or dust-proof) may be used if the staff member is to remain within one metre of the susceptible patient for a period of time. Having the patient wear the mask may save supplies, and give the adult patient some feeling of being in control over the situation. Plastic aprons are used to protect the patient from possible contamination from the staff's clothing or bodies. Aprons may be hung just inside the patient's room and reused for 24 hours, if the outside is wiped each time with a paper towel soaked in a chlorine-based disinfectant and re-hung singly. Material gowns are not waterproof and become progressively more highly permeable to damp and pathogens the longer they are worn. These gowns are only used if a sterile gown is needed to perform an aseptic procedure on a patient.

Linen and waste management

The procedures are similar to the practices that are utilised in all patient care rooms. Colour-coded (e.g. yellow and red) plastic bags are used for contaminated linen and medical waste. Sterilisation of linen is only necessary when a patient is extremely susceptible after bone marrow transplantation or extensive burns. Linen for isolation rooms must be kept as clean as possible and must not be handled by untrained staff, other patients or visitors and may even be stored packed in plastic bags to maintain the highest levels of hygiene. To keep the bioload as low as possible, bedding must be changed every six to twelve hours, and when necessary. Only clean, washed cotton or clean wool blankets received directly from the laundry should be used. Avoid using duvets unless the inners are clean as well, as the fibers can release lint and dust while in use.

Equipment

One thermometer is issued per patient. It is washed after each use and stored dry in a kidney basin/other container in the isolation room. Any equipment needed for more than one patient, such as a blood pressure monitor, must first be washed/disinfected and dried before being taken into the isolation room. Where possible all regularly used items should be dedicated to the isolation area and kept in the patient's room while ensuring that sufficient living space remains for the patient.

Cutlery and crockery

Cutlery and crockery must be washed and stored with the other patients' utensils in the kitchen. If the patient is highly susceptible, his/her cutlery and crockery may be rinsed with boiling water and dried with a clean disposable paper towel, just before serving the meal. Alternatively, disposable plates and cutlery can be used but this may add to feelings of being treated 'differently'.

Bedpans and urinals

If the patient is bedridden or in a single room without a bathroom, a separate bedpan/urinal must be supplied. The bedpan/urinal must be washed and disinfected after each use and stored in the isolation room. Communal bedpans/urinals from the sluice room may be a source of infection for the patient, such as diarrhoea and enteric infections.

Consumable supplies

A small amount of consumable supplies such as adhesive plaster, syringes and needles, alcohol wipes, paper towels, disinfectants, dressings, linen savers, gloves, plastic aprons, caps and masks should be kept inside the patient's room to keep staff from having to leave the room to fetch supplies. Everything needed for isolation must be placed within easy reach just inside the room, to prevent having to go in too

far before putting on the items. Supplies should not be kept in the passage outside the door, because accidental contamination can occur from passers-by or staff who need items quickly.

Plastic locker bags and refuse bin liners

These must be supplied so that the patient can dispose of waste and facial tissues him/herself, as well as to facilitate the swift cleaning of the waste bin and isolation room.

Food and diet

The diet of patients who are extremely susceptible must be monitored to ensure the highest possible level of nutrition without promoting infection through raw or contaminated foodstuffs. Cooked food served warm is preferable to raw, uncooked dishes. Cheese, fermented products such as yeast extract ('Marmite') or ginger ale; fresh salad and fruit such as grapes; yogurt; raw meat such as biltong or smoked sausage, or drinks containing raw egg ('egg flip') can cause infection in highly susceptible patients.

Visitors

Only healthy people old enough to understand the isolation measures should visit an immunosuppressed patient. The staff must watch visitors to ensure compliance with infection control measures. Where the patient is very ill, visitors may be admitted for humane reasons if protective measures are instigated to keep the patient as safe as possible.

Patients who are dying have a particular need for their family or friends to be close by; this should be taken into account and loved ones taught which measures will protect themselves and the patient. If necessary, and with supervision, the patient may be dressed in protective clothing so that visitors may sit on the bed and touch him/her. Visitors must never eat from the patients' plates or drink their drinks and must not be allowed to use the patient's toilet. Hand-washing and disinfection is very important before entering and after leaving the immunosuppressed patients' room.

Pet visitation

In accordance with the Infection Control Department's policy, pet visitation may be allowed, e.g. bringing a well-loved pet to a patient. (Refer to page 226.)

Environmental hygiene

Protective isolation rooms are cleaned first, before the staff undertake any other contaminating jobs. The cleaning staff must use the same protective clothing (e.g. gloves and aprons) as the nursing staff. Their work must be as dust-free as possible, and they must work as quickly as possible. The room must be cleaned with a separate set of cleaning equipment such as a mop, bucket, separate toilet washcloth and duster. After cleaning, the equipment must be removed from the room, washed, dried and stored away from the rest of the ward's cleaning equipment. If necessary, cloths and mop heads may be washed in hot water and dried in the laundry or steam-sterilised in a cardboard box. Permanent cleaners who know the routine should be placed in isolation areas.

Staff health

Only healthy staff should work with immuno-suppressed patients. Skin lesions must be sealed with waterproof plaster or gloves must be worn if the skin of the hands is not intact. Nobody is allowed to work wearing a jersey or woolly garment.

Emotional well-being

Remember that the patient is a person and he/she may become frustrated and tired with being isolated. However, even if one staff member does not comply with the set measures, and breaks the isolation, this makes the efforts of all the other loyal workers worthless. Isolation is 20% hard work and 80% repetition and effort, which can be very traumatic for the patient and the family. Procedures and measures must be applicable to every situation, otherwise they are a waste of time, money and manpower.

Patients in isolation

Objective

Patients who are in isolation receive optimal, holistic care.

If there is any possibility or probability that a patient may be infectious, the appropriate measures must be taken to safeguard the patient, the rest of the patients and the staff against exposure. There must be consensus about the suggested treatment/procedures between the patient, the caregiving staff, the attending doctor, the Infection Control Department and, if necessary, the patient's family – especially if the measures are disruptive.

Isolating patients does not necessarily mean the physical withdrawal of the patient from the previous environment. The patient with a contact transmissible disease may be isolated with relative safety in a general ward, as long as the contact between the patient and the direct environment can be controlled and restricted, e.g. by using occlusive wound dressings to seal the wound. Formidable infectious diseases (e.g. viral haemorrhagic fever or airborne infections such as meningo-coccal meningitis or multi-drug-resistant tuberculosis) rate total isolation and admittance to private rooms where access to and from the patient can be restricted. P4 isolation is the highest level that can be applied.

The caregiving staff and the patient must be kept abreast of the patient's progress. Isolation causes alienation in the patient – especially if visitors are restricted – and the patient soon becomes lonely. A feeling of seclusion and even neglect develops. As long as the patient is informed of the need for the measures and that necessary and specific isolation will make a difference to his/her condition, the procedures become more acceptable. Unfortunately, a very real danger exists that the patient will be neglected, e.g. that cleaning the room will be skipped or dirty linen or crockery will start to pile up. Staff must be aware of this and guard against its happening.

It is quite possible to isolate an infected patient (who cannot be moved) among other patients if the staff employ strict hand hygiene, restrict access to the patient and use protective clothing/equipment.

All staff and visitors that come into contact with an infected patient must follow the prescribed measures if the isolation process is to be successful. Even the smallest breach in the measures may make a mockery of everybody else's effort and spread infection. Staff who are not committed or disagree with the set measures should rather avoid the isolation area and either be moved or be given a different task to perform.

Where possible, staff should be immunised against diseases such as rubella, tetanus and hepatitis B. Immunised staff may still contract the diseases and must take the prescribed precautions, as no immunisation confers total immunity. Immunisation does lessen the acuteness of the disease and most of the damaging long-term side effects of the disease process may be avoided.

The management of waste (including sharps) and linen is discussed in chapter 4. (Refer to pages 152–157 for more detail.)

Prerequisites for isolation

The patient-care area where isolation is to take take place must comply with the following minimum prerequisites:

- The isolation room must contain hand-washing facilities and be well ventilated.

- Unnecessary furniture and equipment must be removed from the room beforehand.
- Sufficient supplies and equipment must be available on hand at the door of the room (e.g. plastic aprons, gloves, masks, caps, plastic bags in the appropriate colours, soap and paper towels, oral thermometers, blood pressure apparatus and any other items needed).
- Prominent signs must be displayed on the door and any other appropriate and visible place to warn uninformed staff of the isolation in progress.
- Thorough records must reflect the progress, continuous holistic care and isolation status of the patient.
- Staff on each shift must be informed about what measures and steps are expected, should an emergency arise. Written infection control measures and precautions, designed with this specific aim in mind should be available.
- The infective patient(s) and/or family must be trained in the type, extent, necessity and fulfilment of the isolation measures before the procedures are set up.
- Pregnant staff must give special attention to the infection control measures and standard precautions to prevent exposure to infection.
- No pregnant staff should routinely care for patients with cytomegalovirus or rubella infection.

Types of isolation

Two types of isolation are generally applied; these are explained below.

1. Source (direct) isolation

This requires measures mainly against contact or airborne conditions. Some authors divide source isolation further into **strict isolation**, **respiratory isolation** and **contact isolation**. This division rests on the method by which the causative organism is transmitted, and what clinical signs and symptoms the patient presents with, so that preventative/control measures may be followed. The principle remains that the method of transfer and the characteristics of the causative micro-organism determine the appropriate measures to be taken. Staff and visitors must use protective clothing and follow specified measures to protect the patient.

Patients are placed in isolation:

- when there is a risk that he/she will spread infection to the staff, other patients or the environment
- if he/she cannot maintain good personal hygiene
- when the patient suffers from an airborne infection
- because of the drug-resistant nature of the micro-organism(s) the patient carries
- when an infected patient is terminally ill and requires constant care and attention

- when there is a risk of environmental contamination by the patient.

2. Protective (reversed) isolation.

Immunosuppressed patients, patients suffering from malignancies such as lymphoma or leukaemia, extensive burn wounds, agranulocytosis, and severe leucopaenia, as well as patients suffering from the loss of extensive skin areas due to wounds or underlying pathology, should all be nursed in protective isolation.

A patient with a white cell count of 200 cells per ml of blood or less is usually considered immunocompromised and is usually placed in isolation to protect him/her against infection.

General measures required for isolation

The following tables indicate when a private room is indicated, and for what conditions.

Table 4.1: Haemorrhagic fever diseases

Indicated for:	Period	Motivation
Lassa fever	Until the urine contains no more virus (± 3 weeks).	Requires P4 isolation followed by room isolation.
Marburg, Ebola and Crimean-Congo fever	Till the platelet count increases and the bleeding stops.	Requires P4 isolation followed by room isolation.
Suspected viral haemorrhagic fevers	Until a diagnosis has been confirmed.	Possible extremely infectious. All staff require protective measures.

Table 4.2: Virulent or highly infectious diseases

Indicated for:	Period	Motivation
Varicella (chickenpox)	For 7 days after the rash appears.	Till the worst of the viraemia is past.
Herpes zoster (shingles)	For as long as the vesicles are present.	Vesicle fluid contains virus and is highly infectious.
Diphtheria	Till 2 successive nasopharyngeal specimens, taken 24 hours apart, culture negative.	Until the period of infectivity passes.
Extensive, infected burns	Until the wounds have healed.	The drainage contains pathogens.

Table 4.3: Immunosuppressive conditions

Indicated for:	Period	Motivation
Extensive, non-infected burns	Until the wounds have healed.	The white cell count is usually low and the patient susceptible to infection, which should be prevented at all costs.
Extensive, non-infected dermatitis	Until the wounds have healed.	The white cell count is possibly low and the patient is susceptible to infection.
Lymphoma, leukaemia, or any patient with a white cell count of less than 200 c/ml	Until the treatment is changed or the white cell count increases.	Until the patient is no longer as susceptible to infection.

Table 4.4: Airborne conditions

Indicated for:	Period	Motivation
Measles	Until 4 days after the rash appears.	Highly infectious. Protection of staff and patients is necessary.
Meningococcal meningitis	Until 24 hours after an appropriate antibiotic has been administered.	As long as viable meningococci are present in the nasopharynx.
Mumps	For 9 days after the glands begin swelling.	Highly infectious in drop form. Patients breathe through their mouths due to the swelling of the nasal passages.
Whooping cough	For 7 days after the rash appears.	For the period of greatest airborne contagion.
Rubella (German measles)	For 5 days after the rash appears.	Highly infectious in drop form. Staff may carry rubella without becoming sick themselves.
Pulmonary tuberculosis/ Multi drug resistant tuberculosis (MDR TB)	2–3 weeks, or until the patient on appropriate/effective drugs responds with clinically observed improvement (e.g. no more pyrexia or night sweats, feels better and coughs less).	Concentrated tuberculosis bacilli in dust are more infectious than organisms in fresh sputum.

Table 4.5: Contact-transmitted diseases

Indicated for:	Period	Motivation
Infected burns	Until fully healed.	Wound drainage may contain opportunistic pathogens.
Gas gangrene	As long as the wound drainage contains viable pathogens and the patient is clinically ill.	Highly transmittable to patients and staff with skin lesions or wounds on the hands.
Herpes zoster (cold sores/blisters)	Until scabs have disappeared.	Scabs contain enervated viral particles.
All exudating wounds, where the patient is mobile, or cannot maintain good hygiene, or the wounds cannot be properly sealed with wound dressing	Until healed.	Wounds may drain through the dressings. Mobile patients with weeping wounds can spread contagion if they use communal bathrooms or lounges.
Any infection caused by drug-resistant bacteria	Until the infection has cleared/no more viable pathogens are present in the lung or wound drainage/ in cultures.	The infection may spread quickly in the patient-care wards due to the fact that antibiotics have very little or no effect on the pathogens.

Table 4.6: Enteric infections

Indicated for:	Period	Motivation
Cholera	For the whole hospital stay.	Prevent any indirect contact with contaminated environments or faeces.
Typhoid	For the whole hospital stay	Prevent any indirect contact with contaminated environments or faeces.
Hepatitis A (suspected or confirmed)	Till one week after the appearance of the jaundice.	Highly infectious between children and persons not maintaining good personal hygiene.
Clostridium difficile	Till three successive stool specimens culture negative.	Very infectious. Complications may have worse side-effects than the disease itself.
Shigellosis/salmonellosis	During the whole hospital stay.	Spreads readily due to poor hand and personal hygiene.
All acute diarrhoea, before a diagnosis is confirmed	Till a diagnosis has been made or three successive stool specimens culture negative.	Due to weakness, frail patients prone to contaminating the environment.
Hepatitis B, C and D in patients without insight into hygienic measures, or who are care-dependent	Entire hospital stay.	Prevent indirect contact with possible contaminated/soiled surfaces or faeces.

Contact isolation

Refer to Table 4.5 above.

Aiborne disease isolation

Refer to Tables 4.1, 4.2, 4.4 and 4.6 above.

Protective isolation

Refer to Table 4.3 above.

Direct (source) isolation

Refer to Tables 4.1 – 4.6 above.

Warning of danger

The universal biohazard danger sign **must be** used to warn staff that an item may be contaminated/soiled with biologically hazardous material. Other possible warning signs include the use of colour-coded plastic bags to seal contaminated/soiled material, as well as the use of special rigid and impermeable containers for contaminated sharp objects such as needles and syringes. In this manner all staff, including external refuse handlers or other illiterate or untrained persons who have to transport the refuse, are warned to be careful.

Access control for infected patients

Access control must be utilised for two reasons: firstly, to ensure the exclusion of people or potential pathogens that can affect the patient's resistance to infection (can transmit infection), and secondly, to protect suscepti-ble people from entering the environment of an infectious person.

Lifting/discontinuing isolation

When the patient's condition no longer warrants continued isolation because any danger to him/herself or the staff/environment has passed, the isolation may be cancelled. In cases of airborne infectious diseases, such as meningococcal meningitis, isolation can be cancelled 48 hours after appropriate treatment with effective antibiotics has been initiated, without the need to repeat a laboratory specimen.

In some cases the recuperating patient remains a source of infection through the presence of enervated organisms, even if the pathogenesis signs and symptoms have started to clear or have completely cleared. Cholera, diphtheria, hepatitis B and C, paratyphoid fever, different forms of pneumonia, rubella, shigellosis, rotavirus diarrhoea, syphilis and herpes simplex stomatitis are some examples of infections that continue to be infectious for a period during the patient's recovery. (Refer to the relevant condition in chapter 2.)

The environment in which the patient was isolated may still be infectious after the patient's recovery and could harbour microorganisms that could become a source of re-infection to the patient or other patients. Staff may also contract infection through handling contaminated equipment or furnishings. Terminal disinfection before reuse of the items will contain the infection.

8 | Special issues

Antibiotic use

Objective

Antibiotics and antimicrobial drugs are used appropriately, while administration is evenly spaced across 24 hours, following the correct route, to ensure effective, stable blood levels.

Definitions

Antimicrobial drugs are compounds that were initially produced after a living organism had been cultured naturally or synthetically in a laboratory, and will inhibit the growth of or kill living micro-organisms including bacteria, protozoa, fungi, and some very simple viruses.

Antibiotics have chemical compounds that are able to kill living susceptible bacteria or interfere with the metabolism of the living organism.

Anti-mycotics are drugs that will inhibit the growth of susceptible fungi or kill them.

Anti-virals are drugs that will inhibit the growth of susceptible viruses.

Anti-protozoal drugs are drugs that will inhibit the growth of susceptible protozoa.

Discussion

Some general antibiotics commonly used are shown in the table below, as well as their usage and general side-effects.

Table 8.1: Antibiotics and their usage

NAME OF DRUG FAMILY	GENERAL USE	GENERAL SIDE-EFFECTS
Penicillin e.g. Cloxacillin, dicloxacillin, methicillin, ampicillin, carbenicillin.	Widely used for treatment of Gram-positive coccal infections, but inactivated by the enzyme penicillinase that is produced by some strains of staphylococcus.	Hypersensitivity reactions such as skin rash, fever, bronchospasm, vasculitis and anaphylaxis are reasonably common side-effects.
Aminoglycoside antibiotics e.g. Gentamycin, amikacin, canamycin, neomycin, streptomycin, tobramycin.	Mostly used for Gram-negative infections.	Erythromycin may cause mild allergies and gastrointestinal discomfort.
Polypeptide antibiotics e.g. Bactracin, colistin and vancomycin.	Effective against severe staphylo-coccal infections and also used in anti-tuberculosis therapy. Colistin or neomyclin is used for diarrhoea caused by Gram-negative enteropathogenic *E. coli*.	Nephrotoxic and ototoxic.

NAME OF DRUG FAMILY	GENERAL USE	GENERAL SIDE-EFFECTS
Tetracycline e.g. Chlortetracycline, minocycline, demeclocycline, doxycycline, oxytetracycline.	Active against a wide variety of Gram-positive and negative micro-organisms and some of the rickettsiae. The antibiotic group is mostly considered bacteriostatic.	Gastrointestinal discomfort, liver- and renal toxicity, photosensitivity. Use of these drugs in the last half of pregnancy until eight years of age may lead to permanent discoloration of the child's teeth.
Kefalosporins e.g. Kefmandole, cefadroxil, cefalexin, cefepime, cefpodoxin.	Resistant against the working of penicillinase. Actively used against infections of the respiratory and urinary tract, middle ear and bone, as well as Gram-positive and negative septicaemia.	May cause nausea, vomiting, diarrhoea, enterocolitis or allergic reactions such as a skin rash, angio-neuritic oedema, or peeling dermatitis. No patient allergic to penicillin must be exposed to kefalosporin.
Choramphenicol e.g. Choramphenicol.	Broad-spectrum antibiotic. Is used less often these days and is usually reserved for patients with acute typhoid fever or severe Gram-negative infections such as *Haemophilus influenzae* meningitis or rickettsiasis.	May cause life-threatening blood abnormalities.

Antibiotic sensitivity tests

Specific sensitivity tests are performed in the laboratory on pure, freshly cultured micro-organisms from patients with infections. The aim is to assess which antibiotics will kill the micro-organisms or at least inhibit their growth until the patient's natural immunity can produce antibodies against them.

Gram colouring is used in the laboratory to make a preliminary identification of the type(s) of micro-organisms in the specimen. After this, the specimen is transferred (planted) from one Petri basin and/or growth medium to the next until a pure colony of one type of micro-organism per basin is cultured. These pure cultures are usually then exposed to Gram-positive and Gram-negative drugs. If the growth of the micro-organism is inhibited by the effect of a specific drug, it is classified as being sensitive to that drug. If the drug has no effect on the growth of the micro-organism, it is considered to be resistant to the drug. The growth can also be non-specific or intermediately sensitive.

The sensitivity assessment usually takes about 48–72 hours to complete, after which the laboratory can indicate which antibiotic will definitely combat the infection. In the meantime, the doctor usually prescribes a general antibiotic to tide the patient over until a specific answer on the therapy is available ('best-chance prescription').

An antibiotic may attack the infecting micro-organism(s) in the patient and start to destroy them, or may support the patient's natural immunity until the body can produce natural antibodies against the infection.

There are different types of antibodies that are all immunoglobulins produced by the lymphocytes in response to penetration of the host's defences by bacteria, viruses or other antigenic (foreign protein) material in the body. An antibody is antigen-specific and will not attack another antigen. The body is able to produce non-specific antibodies on reasonably short notice. These 'general' antibodies will try to phagocytise and control the intruders (antigens) until antigen-specific antibodies can be produced. The healthier and fitter the patient, the sooner this process takes place.

Antimicrobials: administration times

Objective

Antibiotics and other antimicrobials are administered in such a manner that the patient maintains even blood levels across the whole 24 hours of a day.

Development of antimicrobial resistance to drugs

The micro-organisms against which drugs are aimed develop resistance to antimicrobials if the drug doses are not spaced evenly across the whole 24 hours of a day. The micro-organisms multiply during those hours when there is little or none of the drug in the patient's blood circulation, leading to the development of genetic resistance. The resistance is transferred to each of the new generations of micro-organism that develop. When the drug is administered again, the micro-organisms are less sensitive to it. Because the correct dosage of antibiotic has been administered, the weaker micro-organisms will die quickly, but the more resistant ones will keep on multiplying, especially if too many hours pass before the next dose of the drug is administered again. The cycle repeats itself: the sensitive/weaker micro-organisms die from the antimicrobial but the stronger ones keep on multiplying, carrying with them an increasing genetic resistance with each new generation. In the meantime, the patient's own body does not gain the opportunity to produce antibodies against the micro-organisms because they keep on changing, because the drug is being administered, but administered incorrectly.

If time passes in this manner, a severe resistance builds up against the antimicrobial; the patient develops a clinically observable infection due to resistant micro-organisms, which might spread through cross-infection to other patients, the environment or staff. If the cycle is repeated enough times, the micro-organisms become completely resistant to that specific antimicrobial, and possibly to the rest of that family of drugs (drugs which resemble the action of initial drug).

Environmental contamination

If resistant micro-organisms (can) remain viable in the environment, they may become resident (normally found) in a patient-care area or specific department, from where any susceptible patient admitted to the area may be cross-infected.

Combating resistance to antimicrobials

The resistant micro-organisms that remain viable and infect patients will not lose their resistance when a specific antimicrobial is used. Only when the drug is withdrawn from general use does each new generation of that micro-organism become progressively more susceptible to the drug again. This is the reason that restrictions are placed on the general use of certain antimicrobials at times when the medical microbiology laboratory observes that the resistance pattern of micro-organisms found in a hospital or ward is starting to change. The use of these antimicrobials is usually restricted until the micro-organisms regain their normal sensitivity to their use, lifting the antimicrobial pressure on drugs that may lead to resistance of certain micro-organisms.

Chemical interactions

Chemical interactions between antimicrobials and other medications sometimes take place when different drugs are administered to the patient simultaneously. An example is the administration of antacids and oral antibiotics simultaneously. Together they lead to a complex formation – a chemical reaction that stops the antibiotic from being absorbed into the blood stream. In the interim, the infection flourishes uncontrolled – even if the staff administer the drugs on time, following the correct route and dosage.

Administering antimicrobials with food

Usually the pharmaceutical manufacturer specifies if a drug can be administered with food (or a drink such as milk) or not. In some cases food protects the stomach wall against erosion due to the medication, or improves the absorption or effectiveness of the antimicrobial. The two must be given simultaneously.

At other times, a period has to pass before or after the patient has eaten. The administering directions must be followed to ensure the best therapy for the patient. If food is to be taken with the medication, dry biscuits or a piece of fruit should be supplied with the drugs – do not wait to administer the drugs at the regular mealtimes (as these are usually too near to each other in a hospital schedule).

Table 8.2: Schedule for administering any antimicrobials

Administering schedule	Time
Two-hourly (twelve times a day)	06:00; 08:00; 10:00; 12:00; 14:00; 16:00; 18:00; 20:00; 22:00; 00:00; 02:00; 04:00.
Four-hourly (six times a day)	06:00; 10:00; 14:00; 18:00; 22:00; 02:00.
Six-hourly (four times a day)	04:00; 10:00; 16:00; 22:00.
Eight-hourly (three times a day)	06:00; 14:00; 22:00.
Twelve-hourly (twice a day)	10:00; and 22:00; OR 06:00; and 18:00.

Administering antibiotics intravenously

Without exception, small pieces of rubber, air, cotton wool or gauze fibres and even microscopic shards of glass end up in the syringe with which intravenous drugs are administered. If the staff member drawing up the drug does not disinfect the rubber cap of the ampoule beforehand, micro-organisms, dust, other environmental matter and contamination may be administered to the patient during the injection. When giving bolus intravenous injections, foreign matter is injected into the patient's bloodstream, leading to the development of emboli and granulomas in the internal organs. Normally the structure of the syringe is supposed to retain these microscopic objects. If the injection is administered too quickly, the patient might complain of a painful sensation and even perforation of the vein due to expansion with the volume of fluid. Administration as an infusion is a safer method of giving reconstituted antibiotic.

Prerequisites for the infusion of antibiotics

The drug must be freshly reconstituted with the correct solvent (sterile 0,9% saline or sterile water) and added to the fluid in a disinfected vaculiter. The patient's name, the date, the drug, the concentration and time of administration must be written on a label on the bag. The infusion must be completed in the minimum time required.

There are different ways in which antibiotics can be infused:

Added-on lines

- In added-on lines, where a second infusion is connected to the first using a special administering set (a 'Y'), the smaller of the two infusions is placed higher than the other so that gravity will assist the flow of the fluid.
- If fluid flows back from the larger vaculiter via the closed line into the smaller and/or empty one, the smaller vaculiter is hung as high as possible. Do not disconnect the smaller vaculiter. The administering set is always contaminated in this process. Ensure that the patient's arm is immobilised and that the intravenous transfusion device is still correctly positioned in the vein.
- An extension hook is used to lower the main vaculiter below the level of the smaller one while both are in use if the second line does not flow well.
- Added-on lines are changed every 48–72 hours, along with the main set.

Side-lines, connected with a separate needle

- The side-line connected with a sterile needle to the injection port (not the rubber reservoir) of the main line must not be disconnected and hang loose under any circumstances. The open end will be contaminated by dust and micro-organisms from the environment. The infusion fluid remaining in the administering set is quickly colonised by these micro-organisms, which migrate from the contaminated needle upwards into the vaculiter. As soon as a new vaculiter is connected to the contaminated administering set, the organism-loaded fluid is transfused into the patient.
- This side-line's flow regulator is closed and **the whole set is left to hang, still connected to the main line, until the vaculiter is replaced with a new one**. The new vaculiter is simply connected to the set because the needle has remained clean as it has never been removed.
- Side-lines are replaced every 24 hours because they are often exposed to air and environmental micro-organisms.

Antibiotics in side-lines

- Follow the guidelines as discussed under added-on lines.
- In critical care units, where lines are physically removed and often replaced with another administering set and a vaculiter with a new additive, lines are replaced daily unless a special infusion set with needleless injection ports is used. These remain in situ as long as specified by the manufacturer.
- If a vaculiter must be replaced with another one, the used line must be marked with the name of the drug administered through it, the whole set – including vaculiter – must be disconnected from the infusion device (with disinfected or newly washed hands). The hub of the administration set must then be disinfected with 70% alcohol, a sterile injection needle in its sheath connected to the open end to keep the line clean, and the whole unit placed in a clean plastic bag and stored at 4–10°C in the medicine refrigerator until needed again.
- The new vaculiter must be connected to the used administering set, the injection port

of the main line disinfected with an alcohol swab before the cap of the sterile needle can be removed and inserted into the port OR the Luer-lock cap must be disinfected with an alcohol swab, unscrewed and placed in a clean kidney basin, the hub of the Luer-lock disinfected and the administering set connected to it.

Informed consent

Objective

To ensure that patients give informed consent before any procedure is carried out or treatment is administered in the healthcare facility.

Staff must know and be able to apply the following principles:

- Independent, responsible adults have the right to make their own informed choices whether they want to undergo treatment or not, with certain exceptions, for example, if an infection threatens the life of other people. People have, within the law, the right to refuse to be examined, treated or even hospitalised. The parents or guardians of children under the age of independent competence will act on their behalf.
- Persons have the right to culture-specific counselling, preferably in their own language or a common language with the necessary adaptations to make the message clearly understandable.
- 'Admission to a hospital does not imply that the patient has given up the right of security over her/his person. Patients remain persons with the right of control over their own bodies.' (Case of Stofberg v Elliot, 1923.)

Definition of informed consent

Informed consent implies that the legally competent patient will only consent to treatment after he/she has received all the necessary information to enable him/her to choose a course of action.

The elements of informed consent

Informed consent has been given if the patient:

- Clearly understands what the aim of the procedure/examination/intervention is.
- Knows the advantages/disadvantages of the procedure/examination/intervention.
- Knows why the information is required (e.g. a blood test result is needed before surgery can be undertaken).
- Knows what influence the result will have on his/her future treatment.
- Understands how his/her treatment will be adapted/changed by the result of the choice.

Process

- Staff must supply the patient with clear, accurate basic information and must explain further if it is found that the patient has not understood or mastered the information.
- The patient has the right to the truth.
- All possible measures must be taken to assist the patient to understand the information. The use of translators, audio-visual aids and other aids may be necessary.
- If the staff cannot inform or guide the patient properly, this lack of understanding, as well as the measures that were taken in attempting to inform the patient, must be documented in the patient records. Any possible further steps, such as referral to another person, must be taken to ensure that the patient does receive the necessary information.
- A patient may not be tricked or misled into giving consent for treatment.
- Legally, information posters against the wall or pamphlets that describe the procedure/examination/intervention handed over to a patient do not constitute sufficient

pre-test information because of the possibility that the patient may not be able to read or understand what is meant or interpret the meaning of the written words.

- Verbal consent can be obtained from a patient but the healthcare worker must be able to supply proof of this consent. A credible witness must sign the patient's chart to show that they have knowledge of or were present during the information process.
- In the event of injury on duty, or if a staff member has been injured at the bedside during a patient-care procedure, e.g. through a needle prick accident, no blood sample may be taken from a patient without:
  - explaining to the patient why the procedure is necessary
  - counselling them about it
  - gaining consent to the procedure
  - obtaining a signature regarding the process.
- All possible steps must be taken to obtain the patient's informed consent. If the patient refuses after a full explanation and counselling, no blood may be drawn.
- The consent form becomes part of the patient's legal records and must be filed in the chart.

Exceptions to the rule of obtaining informed consent before a procedure/examination/intervention are listed here:

- During a life-threatening emergency to the patient.
- If the patient is unconscious and no blood relative or legal guardian is available to give consent.
- Where the patient has been diagnosed as mentally incompetent and no blood relative or legal guardian is available to give consent.
- Where tests are done on blood donations or for anonymous statistical screening projects.

Consent may be given by any of the following:

- The person who is affected by the procedure.

- All adults who are deemed mentally competent (have the right and ability to make a legal decision), who are sound of mind and not under the influence of any narcotic agent.
- The curator (guardian), legal spouse, parent, child older than 21 years, brother or sister of a mentally ill person.

Note that:

- Married persons must give consent as individuals.
- **Children** older than 14 years may **consent** to their own medical treatment but a parent or guardian remains responsible for contractual arrangements.
- In the case of a child, a caregiver to whom the parent has ceded his/her parental power so that the person may act for the child, usually a family member, or a teacher who cares for the child in the parent's absence.

Legal notification of contagious/infectious diseases

Objective

When a patient or staff member is suffering from a contagious disease, the correct legal and local reporting procedures according to policy are complied with.

Discussion

By law, a number of conditions have been classed as legally notifiable – some due to their infectiousness/risk of transmission and some to evaluate the health status of the community or to give warning that immunisation programmes are not functioning sufficiently. The list of notifiable conditions is periodically updated and published by the Minister of Health in the Government Gazette. (Refer to appendix 1 for the current list.)

In order that timely and appropriate precautionary measures are taken, the Infection

Control Department must be notified of all infectious/transmissible conditions, especially those specified by law. The initial notification is by telephone after diagnosis/admittance.

The treating doctor or registered nurse in charge of the case must report all notifiable diseases in writing as soon as possible after confirmation of diagnosis. The GW 17/5 form must contain a residential address (street address) and be sent to the Infection Control Department, from where it will be sent to the appropriate local authority.

Human rabies, meningococcal meningitis and viral haemorrhagic fevers are the exceptions; as soon as the suspected diagnosis is made, the attending doctor must contact the Infection Control Department, the patient's own referring physician and the Deputy Director of Communicable Diseases in the local Depart-ment of Health, so that the tracing of contacts may begin. As soon as the diagnosis is confirmed, the telephonic message is followed by the GW 17/5 written notification from the attending doctor. (Refer to page 115 for an example of Form GW 17/5.)

The Infection Control Department will assist the patient care area with advice on the necessary isolation measures needed to protect the patient and the staff, if any.

Patient training and education

Objective

Where necessary, a patient and/or his caregiver(s) are taught and trained to care for him either in the healthcare facility or at home. Training and education must become a basic function of all healthcare staff.

Discussion

Patient training is the mutual conferring and receiving of information between the patient and the staff member. The aim is to equip the patient with an understanding of health problems and motivate him/her to take responsibility for his/her own health. The training can be done individually with the assistance of written or audio-visual material, or through the interpersonal intervention of the trainer. Repetition is the key to successful patient education. Often a patient is so ill that he/she cannot understand and therapeutic processes must be continued (even) after discharge. Discharge information strengthens the education the patient has already received, and usually functions as a reference source to assist home adjustment, or remind the patient of what was done or said in hospital.

Guidelines for good patient training

- Start with training at the appropriate time, e.g. as soon after admittance as possible, or after the patient has been diagnosed/mobilised.
- Assess the patient's readiness to learn.
- Plan the contents of the training before the patient, family, staff or attending doctor is approached.
- Collect all possible information and identify the patient's needs before planning the necessary training.
- Consult with other staff involved with the patient to gather as much information about him/her as possible.
- Focus on the patient as the learner.
- Identify the objectives of the training.
- Never force a discussion.
- Devise a patient-care plan or document the training suggestions on an existing plan.
- Involve the nursing staff in evaluating the training given during each shift, in order to adapt the contents as necessary.
- Use the patient's home situation as a background to direct a self-help programme and adapt advice to the circumstances there.
- List the facts one at a time and patiently repeat directions until there is an indication that the patient understands the information.

- Encourage the patient to ask questions.
- Include the patient's social needs or interests in the discussion and inform him/her of community resources that may be available.
- Use fitting language in accordance with the patient's level of education and understanding.
- Listen to the tone of the patient's voice and be aware of any emotional undertones.
- Be aware of the non-verbal body language that may reflect the patient's need for communication (need for touch, a reassuring facial expression, or tone of voice) or negative emotions.
- Discuss family involvement with the patient and choose an appropriate time to involve the family.
- Discuss and/or demonstrate patient-care methods to prevent the spread of infection.
- Remember that if the patient is a child, one or both parents must be present.
- Note that if the patient is dependent on a caregiver, the most appropriate family member must be chosen as the focus of the training, as this person must be able to manage nursing care procedures correctly, and will be able to disseminate information efficiently to any other members of the family.
- Involve a spouse in discussions on hygiene or sexual intercourse.
- Identify potential over-protective family members and counsel where necessary.
- Give support to the family of dying patients.
- Assess the family's understanding and efficiency in patient care, such as the care of infected wounds.
- Refer the family or patient to other appropriate members of the multi-disciplinary patient care team if additional or more specialised information is needed, e.g. a psychologist or psychiatrist.
- Evaluate the patient and/or family's progress in mastering information after each session and before the next session is undertaken.
- Provide discharge advice or information pamphlets to take home and explain the importance of continued self-care at home.
- Document all training and education provided to the patient and/or the family so that there is a permanent record of all the sessions in the patient's file.
- Expect that each session with a patient and/or family will proceed differently due to the individuality of people with differing needs, references, knowledge, fears and strengths.
- Identify each staff member's unique skills, abilities and interests which they utilise when providing training and education. The most suitable person must be identified for each task.

Record keeping

Outcome

Everything that happens to a hospitalised patient during his/her stay in a hospital or healthcare facility is documented and reported.

Objective

That staff take care to fully document all information and details regarding the patient in the hospital chart, including all orders about, observations of, and procedures carried out on and to the patient.

> The golden rule of the South African Nursing Council states clearly:
>
> *If something has not been documented, it has not been done.*

Procedure

Each healthcare worker must take responsibility for patients delegated to his/her care. From the moment of admittance, the staff act as part of a common-law contract with the patient to provide reasonable, meticulous care. The staff member will be held accountable for anything that happens to the patient or that may go wrong. Specific staff members should have delegated tasks that are noted down (e.g. in the attendance register) so that accountability can be determined even after a lapse of time. These records must be kept for a period of 5 years.

The supervising nurse accepts total responsibility for all the patient care while he/she is on duty and must have a synoptic idea of every patient's condition and treatment.

If a patient suffers from an infectious condition, the records must indicate this and detail what interventions the staff have applied to manage the problem. Possible interventions include:

- Whether appropriate isolation measures were implemented in accordance with the route and potential risk of transfer of infection.
- What specific protective clothing and/or equipment was available to protect other patients, staff and the environment.
- In which manner the measures were explained to the patient, the family and other staff members, whether the explanation was understood and which measures were applied to ensure that the information was made clear (e.g. use of an interpreter).
- That all changes in the patient's condition are reflected in the patient's chart and have been reported (what, when, how and to whom should be specified by name).
- Whether treatment given was successful or not, e.g. whether wound drainage was more or less offensive and whether the wound bed was red and viable again after the disin-

fectant used for the wound dressing procedure was changed.
- Whether the safety of the environment was ensured, e.g. a patient with extensive draining wounds was placed in a room with an en-suite bathroom because he/she was weak and could not maintain a good level of personal hygiene.
- That all laboratory results were filed or noted in the patient's records so that all staff members who required the information were able to access it.
- That all reports were dated and legibly signed, and the writer's rank stated.
- That all orders were clearly specified and the results recorded after completion.
- That observations were done on time and accurately documented and signed. Any observed abnormalities (such as pyrexia) were seen as an indication that the time interval between evaluation of vital signs should be speeded up.
- Statements must be motivated and explained. Conduct and actions must be detailed and not just noted, e.g. 'The wound was irrigated with 0,9% saline' rather than just 'wound care done'.
- Time must be specified, e.g. 19:00 rather than 'at night'.
- Incidence reports must be written as soon as possible, and no later than the end of the observer's shift after something extraordinary has happened to the patient, e.g. he developed blisters after a specific antiseptic was used on a wound. The report must be clearly signed by the responsible staff member and verified by the supervisor's signature.
- Only those observations the staff member saw, heard, felt or smelt him/herself should be documented, and not those of any other person, unless specifically required, for example in a psychiatric care setting.
- A healthcare worker must not allow him/herself to be swayed or manipulated

by other staff members to alter any inscriptions in the patient's legal documents. To make false inscriptions is a punishable offence.

Additional information

- Ensure that there is a copy of the infection control policy freely available in the specific patient-care areas to regulate standards of treatment and prevent ignorance/problems.
- The patient must consent to all treatment and procedures before anything is done. If the patient refuses consent for treatment, all possible steps must be taken to change his/her mind. If the patient still refuses, the attending doctor should be informed and the refusal documented in the patient's record.
- Patients and staff all are protected by South Africa's Bill of Human Rights, and this is a handy guideline on the rights of individuals.

Toys and pets

Objective

Staff are able to apply set procedures to protect patients from nosocomial infection through contact with fomites and living surfaces.

All toys are fomites that might harbour micro-organisms, which would allow multiplication and transfer to patients, especially if handled by more than one patient before washing.

Pets can also harbour, transfer, increase or contract infection in a hospital.

Discussion

Toys

- A toy must be cleaned:
  - when it has fallen on the floor
  - before handing it to another child (especially if the first child had it in his/her mouth)
  - if the child that had it last is suffering from a contagious disease/infectious condition/infestation
  - if it is conspicuously soiled.
- Soft, woolly toys should not be allowed in a neonate's hospital crib or cot, as the child is still too small to play with them. Woolly toys are a definite potential source of infection as the items are usually in the way at some time or other and are handled by all staff members, visitors and caregivers.
- Soft toys can be washed with laundry detergent and water if the stuffing is washable. Unwashable soft toys must be commercially dry-cleaned.
- Hospital toys must be washable. Soft, woolly toys may harbour micro-organisms and soon become soiled due to the children's handling of them.
- Wooden toys may splinter and become dangerous, while the rough surfaces are conducive to soiling and harbouring micro-organisms.
- Expensive, soft toys used by a child with a severe infectious disease or contagious condition can be sterilised with ethylene oxide gas but the toy **must be aerated** for at least 4–8 weeks because of the risk of the stuffing retaining the gas, causing fumes that can lead to pulmonary complaints and even skin burns.
- Toys soiled with blood and human body fluids are automatically considered to be contaminated by micro-organisms. They can be carefully rinsed under cold running water, washed in laundry detergent and warm water at a minimum of 65°C, and dried in the sun.
- If it is impossible to wash the toys immediately, they can be wiped with a chlorine-based disinfectant if practical, and allowed to dry spontaneously.
- Unwashable, electronic and very intricate toys are difficult to clean and should rather not be used in a hospital.

Pets

- Pet visitation has singular benefits for a patient who has been hospitalised for a long time, who misses a loved pet badly or who is emotionally depressed. Although there are a lot of benefits, there are as many problems to this procedure.
- Pets should only be allowed in a hospital if the attending doctor and the Infection Control Department know about the visit, have given permission and co-ordinate the process.
- Pets are not allowed to visit a patient who has a contagious disease that the animal can contract, e.g. diarrhoea.
- Strict supervision must be kept and no other patient or staff member should be allowed to play with or have access to the animal.
- Pets must be clean, healthy and non-infested before they are allowed to visit a patient.
- The patient should be accommodated separately, preferably in a single room with the door closed.
- The person who brings the pet must ensure that it does not run around the hospital and must clean up after the animal if it should make a mess.
- The patient must wash his/her hands well after the visit. A bath and a change of nightclothes afterwards are indicated, if the patient is able to manage this.
- If the 'pet' is an aquarium of fish in the room, the water in the tank must be changed every second day by the staff or a visitor. Care should be taken that the patient has no contact with the used water, which must be discarded down the sanitary sewer.
- Chickens and birds often carry loose parasites on their feathers and should preferably not be allowed in a hospital.

Visitors

Objective

No visitor is exposed to infection or contributes to infection in the healthcare setting. Staff must understand that visitors play a small but important role in the spread of infection, and careless or exposed visitors may easily spread contact and airborne conditions. Staff must be able to apply procedures to minimise these risks.

Procedure

Here are some suggestions to ensure safe visiting:

- No sick person should be allowed to visit a patient, especially a visibly infected visitor suffering from any form of upper respiratory infection, fever, influenza, herpes zoster, gastroenteritis or a skin rash of uncertain origin.
- Visitors should be taught to wash their hands before and after visits to patients in isolation rooms, as well as those suffering from weeping wounds, a skin rash and/or a productive cough.
- Visitors to patients in respiratory or strict isolation should be limited. No children younger than thirteen should be allowed without consulting the staff. Young children are a frequent source of infection and are also prone to acquiring infection due to their developing immunity.
- The nursing staff should supervise people visiting patients in isolation in order to limit the risk of exposure to infection(s).
- Visitors must be prevented from carrying their belongings into an isolation room as this promotes the spread of infection. If an item has to be taken in for safety's sake, it is sealed in a clear plastic bag that can be washed off or discarded at the end of the visit. The bag must not be opened inside the isolation room. If this does happen, the

item must remain inside the room or be washed/disinfected before removal.

- Visitors who assist with patient care (such as mothers in paediatric wards) must be taught how to assist and what they may/can do and their skill must be checked before the nursing staff relax their supervision.
- Cross-infection with community- or hospital-acquired micro-organisms will be promoted if visitors are allowed to sit on the patient's bed or an empty bed, or when they place personal belongings or bags on these surfaces. At the same time, visitors should not be allowed to use the patients' eating utensils, linen (especially towels) or toilet facilities.
- Visibly unhygienic visitors or persons with obviously soiled clothing or bodies should be informed very diplomatically that they will not be allowed to visit the patient in such a condition – especially if the patient is resident in a general ward.

- Pet visitations are only allowed under strict supervision and in accordance with the individual circumstances in each patient's case. Sick, neglected or dirty animals will not be allowed to 'visit' patients. (Refer to page 227.)
- Blind persons' guide dogs are allowed inside the hospital as they are considered to be visual aids rather than pets.

Some areas where access should be controlled or visitors may need to be limited/excluded:
- critical care units
- maternity suites
- operation theatres and recovery rooms
- neonatal/baby units
- special paediatric critical care areas
- the rooms of patients in protective (reversed) isolation
- areas where visitors are prohibited on request of the patient or attending doctor.

Children of healthcare workers with infectious conditions

Objective

No patient or staff member is exposed to infection. Staff whose children have infectious conditions discuss the situation with their supervisor as soon as possible.

Discussion

If the staff member maintains good personal hygiene and washes his or her hands when coming on duty, the chances of transmitting contact-borne infection to the work area is statistically small.

The parents or caregivers of children with airborne infections may become temporary carriers of the causative micro-organism(s) or other pathogens as the organisms are inhaled and sheltered in the nasopharynx. Usually these 'foreign' organisms are eradicated from the body within 48 hours by the host's normal body flora, unless there is continuous or regular contact with the source (the sick child).

Staff with sick children should explain the situation to their supervisors at work, so that the infection risk can be assessed and monitored. If necessary, the parent might have to attend an occupational health clinic or visit her/his own physician to obtain prophylaxis against possible infection.

Exposure on duty (splashes in the face/exposure to possible infectious material/patients)

Objective

Staff exposed to infection must be assessed and treated, if possible. Staff members who have definitely or potentially been exposed to infective material or patients report the exposure or incident immediately so that the risk can be assessed and further action taken.

Procedure

- The staff member must report the incident immediately or as soon as possible before the end of the shift to the direct supervisor.
- Report the incident telephonically to the infection control staff, including all the relevant information such as:
  - the clinical diagnosis and condition of the patient, e.g. terminally ill with hepatitis B infection
  - the character of the exposure (e.g. contact with blood, splashes of blood and human body fluids in the eyes, or contact with a suspected or confirmed droplet or airborne disease such as tuberculosis or meningococcal meningitis)
  - what was done after the incident to control the exposure or to correct the incident, e.g. whether the splattered eyes were rinsed out with sterile saline.
- The necessary referrals and arrangements must be made in accordance with each individual incident.

- If the staff member is to receive post-exposure prophylaxis (e.g. antibiotics or anti-retroviral therapy), the Emergency Room staff, Infection Control Department and/or Occupational Health Department should organise this.
- The Emergency Room's doctor should assess whether the staff member qualifies to receive chemo-prophylaxis and should prescribe the medication/drugs. The exposed staff members must be listed on a medicine prescription chart and the appropriate drugs prescribed (either as a written or telephonic prescription – telephonic prescriptions must be confirmed in writing as soon as possible).
- The medication must be made available and the necessary information regarding administering the prophylaxis given individually to the exposed staff members, or each may collect the medication and information from the pharmacy themselves. Receipt of the medication must be signed on the prescription chart, after which the chart must be sent to the Occupational Health Clinic for filing.
- Any side-effects, or signs and symptoms of illness must be reported immediately to the Occupational Health Clinic.
- The exposure history and prophylactic intervention must be noted in each staff member's file, as must any refusal to accept treatment/untimely discontinuance of treatment.

Injury on duty, exposure on duty, sharps-related injuries, needle-prick accidents

Objective

Staff exposed to an injury on duty (IOD) report the incident immediately and follow set procedure as prescribed, so as to prevent incident-related infection.

Proposed policy/procedure regarding exposure to HIV/AIDS infection

Weekdays

- Report the incident immediately to the direct supervisor.
- Report to the Emergency Room or Occupational Health Clinic so that a blood sample can be taken, and complete the necessary injury on duty reports.
- The staff member must receive pre-test counselling and then must give permission to draw blood for laboratory HIV and hepatitis B (HBV) analysis.
- The blood sample and the completed request forms must be sent to the virology laboratory.
- The Emergency Room or Occupational Health Doctor must evaluate the staff member's exposure risk and prescribe either single, double or triple prophylactic anti-retroviral therapy or decide that no treatment is necessary, either by telephone or as a written prescription.
- The necessary injury on duty forms must be completed:
  - report of an IOD
  - statement about an IOD
  - supervisor's declaration
  - physical assessment or trauma record from the Emergency Room/Occupational Health Clinic.
- An appointment must be made to see the appropriate doctor for a first medical assessment, as well as a date when the blood results will be given during post-test counselling.
- The staff member must be evaluated in regard to the need for prophylactic treatment and a prescription issued.
- The staff member takes the prescription to the appropriate pharmacy for the medication. Either all or part of the medication can be issued, e.g. the pharmacist may issue just

enough for a week to ensure that the staff member can continuously be evaluated when they return for the rest of the prescription.

- The first dose must be taken immediately (preferably within 1–8 hours after exposure.)
- Follow-up appointments are made for assessment after three months, six months or twelve months, if relevant, by the Emergency Room or Occupational Health Clinic, after which the final medical assessment can be completed.

Treatment

- If the staff member is HIV-negative and the source patient is HIV-positive, the staff member may be treated with single, double or triple therapy, according to the exposure risk and the doctor's preference.
- If the source/original patient involved in the injury is unknown, the staff member should be treated as if the source has tested HIV-positive.
- If the staff member is found to be HIV-positive, no treatment is given, but the staff member is counselled regarding future choices of treatment.
- If both the staff member and the source patient have tested HIV-negative, the staff member is counselled to go for follow-up testing (because of the influence of the HIV-'window period').
- If the staff member tests HBV-negative, he/she must be immunised against hepatitis B according to the set policy and administering schedule.
- If the staff member tests HBV-positive, no further treatment is administered but the staff member is counselled accordingly.

After hours and on public holidays

- Report the incident immediately to the direct supervisor.
- Report to the Emergency Room to draw blood for HIV and HBV and to complete

the first injury on duty reports (refer to the 'Weekdays' section on page 230).

- The staff member receives pre-test counselling and then gives permission to draw blood for HIV and HBV analysis.
- The blood sample, together with the completed request forms, are sent to the laboratory, where they are stored until the next work day.
- The Emergency Room doctor assesses the patient's exposure risk and prescribes single, double or triple therapy on the staff member's casualty chart.
- The Emergency Room staff request the emergency issuing of medication, which the staff member personally receives, together with the necessary information regarding the therapy.
- The first dose must be taken immediately (within 1–8 hours maximum after exposure, to ensure optimum therapeutic blood levels).
- The staff member must visit the Occupational Health Clinic on the next working day to ensure that the documentation is in order, that everything has been completed correctly and that the correct blood specimens have been taken. The laboratory results must be made available or an appointment made for the results to be given. The results should always be given personally during the first medical assessment or at a special post-test counselling interview.
- The staff member makes follow-up appointments at the Occupational Health Clinic for three months, six months and twelve months (as appropriate), after which the final medical assessment will be completed.
- For treatment, refer to the section above.
- The Occupational Health Doctor must complete a (written) prescription that can be sent to the pharmacy to replace the temporary casualty prescription.

After-hours emergency testing

Sometimes blood analysis has to wait; possibly until a day shift comes on duty in the laboratory, or a suitably qualified technologist becomes available. Chemo-prophylactic treat- ment can be started immediately after exposure to infection, even without a blood analysis. If the prophylactic treatment is unnecessary, it can simply be stopped and the issued medication returned to the pharmacy or discarded. (Please refer to the diagram below.)

Diagram of actions to be taken after occupational exposure to HIV/HBV

INJURED SOURCE:

*PEP =
Post-Exposure
Prophylaxis

Immediate actions

- Let wound bleed/squeeze blood from needle prick
- Wash with warm water and soap
- Disinfect with disinfectant or 70% alcohol
- Report to the immediate supervisor
- If the source's viral status is unknown try to obtain blood from source (informed consent) or treat as if positive.

Weekdays	After hours/public holidays
1. Report to the Occupational Health Clinic	1. Report to the Emergency Room
2. Counselling of the injured	2. Counselling of the injured
■ HIV	■ HIV
■ HIV testing	■ HIV testing
■ Possible post exposure prophylactics (PEP)	■ Possible post-exposure prophylactics (PEP)
3. Draw blood for HIV/HBV studies and send it to virology	3. Draw blood for HIV/HBV studies and store it in laboratory until next working day.

THE HIV LAB TEST COULD BE DONE AS AN EMERGENCY TEST

If positive:

- PEP SHOULD BE CONTINUED
- MONITORING SHOULD CONTINUE AS STIPULATED IN THE DOCUMENT

If negative:

- STOP PEP, OR CONTINUE TO COMPENSATE FOR A POSSIBLE WINDOW PERIOD

The transmission of HIV/HBV

1. The average risk of infection from all types of percutaneous exposures to HIV infected blood is 0.3% and for HBV the risk is 9–35%. Only blood and sexual fluids are contagious and not faeces or urine unless it is contaminated with blood
2. Zidovudine, singly and/or in combination with lamivudine, when given within 8 hours following exposure has been shown to be 97% effective in preventing seroconversion.
3. Please make sure that all procedures are followed according to the official guidelines to ensure that the PEP is taken in good time.
4. High-risk exposure would entail the following and PEP should be recommended:
   - a deep injury
   - the presence of visible blood on the device
   - injury with a needle that has been placed in a vein or artery
   - high viral load in source patient (terminally ill patient who dies within 60 days of the episode or a patient in the seroconversion phase).

Management of sick staff

Objective

For all staff to be aware that the policy on the management of sick staff rests on the prevention of cross-infection spreading from the staff to the patients (or back) as well as limiting the development of infection.

In principle, acutely ill staff are not supposed to report for duty or remain at work. Staff who are not contagious and are able to work whilst unwell may do so, applying the strictest possible infection control and prevention measures. Staff on duty who are sick must report to their direct supervisor and if necessary visit a doctor or attend the Occupational Health Clinic if the symptoms persist. Staff who are suffering from any respiratory, skin or enteric (diarrhoeal) condition and have direct contact with patients or food, should be excused from duty as soon as possible.

Staff with chronic conditions such as asthma, unhealed leg ulcers, shingles, asymptomatic HIV infection (or AIDS), eczema or any other condition that is not directly transmissible to other persons in the workplace, may work with the permission of the supervisor. It is preferable that they be placed in work areas that offer some protection to themselves, the patients and other workers. All possible infection control measures must be taken, e.g. leg ulcers must be covered with occlusive dressings that are not removed during the time at work. In practice it is not always so easy to keep to this principle. The following measures are suggested to prevent the spread of infection should sick staff be forced to report for duty.

Procedure

Report these conditions to the staff member's supervisor or the Infection Control Department:

- Acute diarrhoea with symptoms such as fever, abdominal cramps, bleeding or diarrhoea lasting longer than 24 hours.
- Herpes simplex of the mouth and face.
- Herpatic whitlow of the nails.
- Diagnosed *Streptococcus pyogenes* (group A) sore throat.
- Infected skin lesions, especially on exposed skin areas.
- Acute upper respiratory infection or severe influenza.
- Active infection after exposure to:
  - conjunctivitis (including 'pink eye')
  - diphtheria
  - hepatitis
  - herpes simplex virus (cold sores) (if not immune)
  - human immunosuppressive virus
  - measles (if not immune)
  - mumps (if not immune)
  - polio and/or acute flaccid paralysis
  - rubella (if not immune)
  - tuberculosis
  - varicella zoster virus (chickenpox/shingles) (if not immune);
  - any other disease that the staff member is not immune to or to which he or she has been exposed (e.g. meningococcal meningitis).

These notifications must be followed up individually and managed accordingly. Where the situation dictates or exposure to a confirmed disease has taken place, the appropriate treatment/prophylaxis should be given. Staff with contagious conditions should be excused from duty until the condition has cleared.

Staff who suffer from any of the listed conditions or who could have been exposed to them are referred to the appropriate discussions in chapters 2 and 3 of this book for information on work/school exclusion, etc. Staff suffering from minor ailments that develop while on duty should report to the

Occupational Health Clinic during weekdays or at the Emergency Room after hours to have their complaints seen to.

Contact-transmissible infectious conditions

Examples include: wound sepsis, conditions characterised by fluid-filled vesicles (e.g. chickenpox, herpes zoster and herpes simplex type II), patients with full-blown AIDS, impetigo, staphylococcal or streptococcal skin infection, viral haemorrhagic fevers. To a lesser extent, infestation with lice and scabies is also contact-transmissible although longer and more direct contact with linen and affected persons is required for this to take place.

If the staff member is able to physically work without becoming a threat to the patients, other staff or the environment, he/she may work as long as:

- The condition is not too extensive or severe.
- The wounds are starting to heal.
- No contaminating external leakage of wound drainage takes place and the wound is sealed with an occlusive dressing. No wound care may be done at work except if the staff member attends a clinic service such as the Occupational Health Clinic or a polyclinic while on duty.
- The staff member is responsible for, and will keep up, the preventive measures even when the wounds begin to heal.
- The staff member has been on effective antimicrobial treatment for longer than 48 hours – a registered doctor must prescribe the treatment. (This is not appropriate for all the listed conditions).
- The attending doctor has no objections.
- The staff member has no direct/indirect contact with patients or food (e.g. cleaning patient-care equipment or working in the pharmacy).

Airborne infectious diseases

Some examples include: chickenpox, herpes zoster and herpes simplex type I stomatitis, measles (rubeola), diptheria, meningococcal meningitis, meningococcaemia, mumps, whooping cough, rubella, respiratory tuberculosis, haemophilus influenza epiglottis, severe influenza and the common cold.

No staff member with an infectious respiratory condition may report for duty, as there is no faultless or perfect method of controlling the spread of micro-organisms. The safest course is for the staff member to remain at home.

Enterically transmitted infectious diseases

Some examples include: salmonellosis (including typhoid), cholera, viral and bacterial shigellosis, gastroenteritis and hepatitis A.

Staff with diarrhoea should not deliver direct or indirect patient care, or have contact with food until the condition has cleared. The staff member must know that the stool may still contain causative micro-organisms for a week after the last episode of diarrhoea. Good hand hygiene is essential as well as a high level of environmental hygiene and sanitation to prevent the spread of infection.

Staff who are not contagious and remain on duty should take special care about applying hand hygiene and avoid giving direct patient care.

Management of a colleague who is HIV-positive

Your colleague will probably be experiencing many of the following after exposure to HIV:

- Anxiety followed by severe depression.
- Fear of the unknown, and fear of the laboratory results. The colleague could initially attempt to suppress the fear and will repeatedly analyse the exposure, the extent of the incident as well as the risk of infection to the rest of the family.
- Selectivity about how and when the incident

will be made known to others. People are usually very reticent about what happened and will keep quiet and endure the uncertainty alone if any blame can be attached to their own actions.

- Loss of concentration and perhaps becoming neglectful or over-cautious.
- Some or all of the six stages of bereavement: shock and disbelief, denial, anger, bargaining, depression and acceptance, in the same manner as any other person who receives bad news.

The colleague will attempt to give meaning to what has happened or to rationalise it.

They will experience a need to start working through the possibility of severe illness, future physical mutilation and even the possibility of death. They may start to blame the source patient and question the meaning of their work/profession.

The staff member should be handled with patience, support, understanding and care. This person may be very unpredictable and fragile for the next few months until the last of the blood tests have been completed and the results are known.

Hints on how to handle someone who has been exposed to HIV infection or is HIV-positive:

- Do not demand that the person should tell you what is wrong with him/her.
- Consider the information confidential if he/she does tell you.
- Do not give advice unless asked.
- Before saying or asking anything, find out what the colleague thinks.
- Be a friend – give support.
- Be culture-sensitive.
- Do not tell jokes about HIV/AIDS in public.
- Accept the person and respect the human being, even if their behaviour is unacceptable.
- Remember that AIDS generates fear, often regarding the person's own mortality and possible sexual behaviour.
- Remember that AIDS sufferers and HIV-positive persons have the same rights as all other people, as well as the usual obligations to their fellow human beings.
- Protect your colleague: encourage the use of protective barriers and clothing under all circumstances and do not consciously expose the person to known infection.
- Accept that the colleague's immunity is not as strong as that of others and that he/she will experience more complaints of illness, or will be absent from work more often.
- Remember these two principles: the 'need to know' and 'obligation to warn'. Both must be employed with care and good judgement. Always ask 'Who needs to know?' and 'Who am I obliged to warn?' before saying anything about the colleague's condition.

Psychological management of staff who are HIV-positive or living with AIDS

These colleagues will require:

- Individual professional counselling on how to adapt practise and work to avoid cross-infection.
- Support from colleagues.
- Knowledge of, and skill in the use of, protective clothing, other barriers (such as mouth-to-mouth airways and resuscitation bags) and techniques (such as the creation of a neutral area in an operating theatre in which to hand over sharp instruments).
- A non-judgmental working environment in which the staff member can speak of fears and confront irrational thoughts without fear of reprisal.
- Support groups, e.g. other persons living with AIDS or who are HIV-positive.

These colleagues must **avoid** the following:

- Radical decision-making. Shortly after diagnosis there is a period of uncertainty about everything in their private lives. Situations during which decisions must be made (e.g. whether they will have treatment) or discussions about AIDS, cause feelings of helpless exhaustion.

- Any situation in which the sufferer will be exposed to someone else's blood or an infection risk, as well as procedures that carry additional risk, such as:
  - suturing wounds in hollow structures, e.g. an episiotomy (where the person's fingers are out of sight in a small enclosed area in the presence of a sharp instrument
  - orthopaedic operations where there are sharp bone ends
  - the palpation of sharp instruments (e.g. the blades of a pair of scissors in a body opening)
  - any other penetrating (invasive) procedures.
- Physical contact with patients, contaminated linen or instruments if the skin of the hands is broken
- Contact with physically ill patients, especially those with confirmed highly infective diseases such as measles or chickenpox
- Unsafe sexual practices (e.g. violent sex; anal sex; unprotected sex; sex with unknown persons or sex under the influence of drugs or alcohol).
- Pregnancy, taking into account the viral load in the person's blood as well as the immunosuppressive stage in which the person is at present.

Staff health programme/occupational health/pre-employment evaluation of staff health

Objective

That only healthy staff members work with patients, and for staff to be informed about

the staff health programme. A staff health programme is part of the total infection control programme of the hospital/healthcare facility complex. Information on the programmes must be available to all staff members. Staff need to be healthy themselves in order to deliver optimal patient care.

Objectives of the programme

- The initiation and maintenance of high standards of personal hygiene and responsibility for individual infection control practices among the staff.
- Surveillance and investigation of infectious conditions, possible exposure to contagious conditions and outbreaks of infection among staff in co-operation with the Occupational Health Department.
- Treatment of staff with work-related infectious conditions or exposure.
- Identification of work-related infective conditions and the implementation of appropriate preventive/control measures.
- Identification of unnecessary procedures that may give rise to greater financial expense to the healthcare institution.
- The implementation of interventions to reduce/prevent the absence/disability of the staff due to infectious conditions.
- Prevention of morbidity and mortality due to infectious conditions among the staff.

Procedure

- Staff health and safety education must be provided during the post-appointment orientation and provided/reinforced by continuous in-service training.
- The hospital/healthcare facility's infection control guide must be available in each department, and contain policy on patient care procedures, staff safety and environmental hygiene.
- Work-related infectious conditions and exposure must be investigated and referred

to the Occupational Health Department for follow-up/documentation, or can be managed by the Infection Control Department.

- The Infection Control Committee co-ordinates planning and administration on health policy and procedures in the hospital/healthcare facility in order to take into account the administrative and patient-care functions of the institution.
- The infection control surveillance programme is directed at the notification of infectious conditions as prescribed by law, as well as the identification of conditions that require the work exclusion or limitation of staff, and any epidemiological investigation or contact tracing that may be required.
- Occupational health officers are represented on the Infection Control Committee to simplify co-operation and co-ordination.
- The Occupational Health Department undertakes pre-employment screening.

Personal hygiene, clothing and jewellery

Objective

For staff to be aware of, and able to apply, the policies and procedures concerning personal hygiene, in order to maintain high infection prevention and control standards at all times.

Procedure

Staff members must wear clean uniforms each day as the contact with the micro-organisms from the patients and hospital/healthcare facility/home environments leads to immediate and unavoidable colonisation of material.

Uniforms/clothing

Within six hours after leaving home and reporting for duty (already carrying a number of micro-organisms), the clothing of staff members will bear a representative sample of all the micro-organisms of the patients, the other staff members and the environment. These micro-organisms are continually exchanged (disseminated) to and from patients, colleagues and the environment. If the same clothing is worn again the next day, this heavy load of micro-organisms (bioload or bioburden) is still present and only increases.

Hands

Because the person has contact with her/his clothing, micro-organisms are unavoidably transferred to their hands and the rest of their skin, and from there to other persons and surfaces. Cross-infection is advanced without the person even being aware that he/she is a source of infection.

Sitting on beds

Due to the bioload that clothing carries, no-one should sit on a patient's bed or on an unoccupied bed. The micro-organisms deposited can lead to infection of the (next) resident of the bed.

Hair and skin

In reality, human hair is a continuation of the dry layers of the epidermis. The same micro-organisms that appear on the skin will be present in the hair, but in greater numbers. The skin is washed more often than the hair, with the result that the micro-organisms multiply undisturbed in the hair (and in the beards of males). If the head is contaminated with hospital- (or other healthcare facility) acquired micro-organisms, the person's hands will be contaminated as soon as he/she scratches the scalp or touches the hair.

When patients/staff shout, cry, cough or even speak, micro-organisms are set free from the airways and will spread between 1–2 m, splattering over other staff members and the environment. The drops cling to the staff member's face and hair, dry out, splinter off and are deposited on the face and hands as soon as the person looks down to see what he/she is doing. In this manner washed hands and sterile work surfaces are unknowingly contaminated with drops, loose hair, dry dust particles containing the nuclei of micro-organisms and skin flakes (which can carry up to 100 000 staphylococci per layer). When aseptic procedures are performed, a clean paper cap should be worn, covering all the hair. The cap is exchanged as soon as the procedure is completed, or if it becomes damp or tears. For the remainder of the time it is left untouched. The wearer's hands are contaminated if he/she constantly fusses with the cap. Hands should be washed after contact with a used cap.

Nails

Nails should never be longer than medium length because patients and colleagues can easily be scratched when a patient in a damp bed is lifted or turned. Scratches usually become infected due to the large number of micro-organisms that are present in the warm, moist and contaminated areas under the nails.

Nail polish protects the surface of the nail, but disinfectant and antiseptic soap dry it out and causes it to splinter off, leaving the nail thinner than usual. Fungi and bacteria can penetrate the cracks in and around the nail bed and lead to infections that are difficult to cure. Small flakes of nail tissue and nail polish can be deposited as foreign objects in wounds or on sterile areas. 'Gel' and false nails can harbour fungi, although heat-laminated nails are less prone to this problem.

For safety's sake, staff members should never bite or chew their nails while on duty, or eat in a patient-care area without first washing their hands with soap and water.

Rings and wristwatches

Rings and wristwatches create warm, moist and contaminated areas in which micro-organisms can multiply undisturbed, because soap and water never reach them. Rings with inset stones may injure the skin of patients and colleagues. All rings, including plain wedding bands and wristwatches, must be removed when a staff member scrubs for an aseptic procedure. Chemical reactions between the soap, the disinfectant and the metal of jewellery can cause severe dermatitis or eczema that may leave wounds or lesions on the hands or forearms of staff members. In time, the mechanism and surfaces of watches and rings are damaged by glove powder and chemical reactions.

Refer to page 20–23 for a more detailed description of the protective clothing that is available to protect staff against contamination and possible contagion.

Staff development and training

Objective

Healthcare staff must be correctly trained and must understand that training is a fundamental task and responsibility of everyone working in the healthcare environment.

Procedure for staff training

Staff training is provided on three levels:

Informal – one-on-one training, e.g. when patient-care areas are visited and the staff are spoken to.

In-service training, e.g where there is a specific problem in an area and staff are trained to solve or prevent the problem or if organised workshops are held.

Formal training in a classroom set-up, e.g. staff development lectures or continuous training work assignments.

Basic skills of a trainer

Basic affective skills

- Use an individual approach for every patient/staff member.
- Keep eye contact with patients or students when speaking to them. Remember that in some cultures, the person who is sub-servient and who wants to show respect for a trainer will not make continuous direct eye contact with him or her. This respect-ful person is listening and not ignoring the speaker.
- Maintain professional conduct.
- Consider your own responses to the patient's conduct during training.
- Take responsibility for your own decisions.
- Allow the patient or student to verbalise or express fear.
- Wait during silences in interviews for the other person to take the lead in the conver-sation – do not be intimidated by silence.
- Manage stressful situations as early as pos-sible, before they spiral out of control.
- Handle aggressive patients and learners appropriately and as early as possible to prevent future interruptions.
- Maintain good working relationships and co-operation with all staff and doctors, as they will evaluate what you are striving for and have achieved .

Basic cognitive skills

Assessment skills

- Identify the character of the patient, his strengths and weaknesses.
- Identify the counselling needs in the learner and family.
- Assess the patient's immediate emotional status.
- Adjust to the immediate situation.
- Talk to the learner in a relaxed manner.
- Make use of an interpreter or adjust to a learner with a language problem, or a dis-ability such as blindness or deafness.

- Assess the learner's need for referral to another patient-care service or medical discipline.
- Assist staff in patient-care areas to assess the specific needs for special attention of a dependent or independent patient in isolation.
- Assess and observe any causal factors lead-ing to problems in a learner.
- Assess the need for follow-up visits or fur-ther counselling in a learner.
- Adjust the environment to the needs of the patient, e.g. acquiring a special chair or bed for someone who is very tall or who cannot sit or stand for long.

Educational (training) skills

- Plan and implement training programmes.
- Set goals for learners that can be evaluated.
- Use visual and audio-visual aids in teach-ing, e.g. pamphlets, videos and audio cas-settes.
- Ask questions and encourage participation in training to gauge the level to which the learner has mastered the teaching material.
- Adjust language to the learner's level of understanding.
- Summarise the contents of the session at the conclusion of the lesson.
- Be aware of medical and legal factors that may influence the training.
- Inform the learner of any community resources or sources of support that he/she may later access.
- Evaluate, on a continuous basis, the efficacy of every facet of training and adjust to cir-cumstances if the patient does not achieve the necessary level of proficiency or progress.
- Train the staff in the patient-care areas and support services in aspects of patient and personal infection control and safety.

Administrative skills

- Liaise with the staff in patient-care areas on the training of the patient.

- Compile reports on the progress of the staff and patient(s) after training.
- Evaluate training and education against a measuring instrument to assess efficacy/re-plan.
- Undertake inspections as necessary.
- Identify and undertake interventions to correct problems in the staff, patient or environmental infection control system.

Staff immunisation

Objective

As part of the hospital/healthcare facility's infection control programme, as well as the legal responsibility of the institution to protect its staff from exposure to disease, all newly appointed staff are immunised as far as possible against the major infectious diseases found in the facility.

Procedure

- New staff should undergo a pre-employment medical examination and physical assessment at the Occupational Health Department.
- The following immunisation is often done routinely:
  - a tetanus toxoid booster dose is administered if the staff member has not been immunised during the past ten years
  - hepatitis B immune status analysis and/or vaccination for all medical and paramedical staff who have contact with blood and blood-products, as well as specified housekeeping staff, patient porters and security staff
  - rubella vaccine for maternity departments' staff, if the blood titre level of the

staff member is low or does not indicate immunity
  - appointed staff may require further immunisation if exposed to certain infectious diseases such as diphtheria, measles, whooping cough or polio.
- Because of contact with sick patients, staff may require specific prophylaxis that is not covered by immunisation, e.g. antibiotics after exposure to meningococcal meningitis or pulmonary tuberculosis. This type of prophylaxis is usually given in conjunction with the Infection Control Department and the Occupational Health Clinic.
- Further tests may be indicated by clinical evaluation and the staff member's medical history, e.g. sputum analysis can be done after specific complaints of night sweats, cough, and weight loss.
- Staff with tuberculosis-positive sputum smear cultures must be referred to a primary health clinic for treatment and follow-up if the diagnosis has been confirmed, or while they are awaiting the final diagnosis.
- On appointment and annually thereafter, catering staff may be required to provide a stool specimen for laboratory analysis (including microscopy, culture and parasite studies). If a caterer or food handler complains of illness or symptoms such as upper respiratory disease or diarrhoea, he/she must immediately report to the Occupational Health Clinic for assessment and/or treatment.
- Staff with complaints of infectious conditions that cannot be treated as minor ailments at the Occupational Health Clinic must be referred to or make an appointment to see their own general practitioner/ private physician.

10 | Infection control in home-based care settings

Introduction

Patients cared for at home often have the benefit of being in an area of low infection risk, as they are used to the micro-organisms in their own environment, their family members and regular caregivers. Often patients are more relaxed and less confused at home and may feel that they have retained a measure of choice and control over their own lives. This should improve their inherent immunity as the stress of being in a strange environment is reduced.

There is a potentially negative aspect to home-based care: if an immune-compromised patient (such as one living with a life-limiting disease) is released from a healthcare facility with a communicable nosocomial infection that clinically presents only when the person reaches home, there is then a risk that the infection can be transmitted to caregivers.

From the caregiver's side, an occupationally acquired infection may cause temporary or even permanent disability and disease, affecting the caregiver as well as their family. Therefore a patient with a transmissible infection will need to take more thorough prevention measures than one whose condition is not contagious, e.g. a patient suffering from tuberculosis must adjust his/her usual way of coughing and disposing of coughed-up sputum. This can be achieved mainly through application of a standard programme of infection prevention and control practice by caregivers that will lead to a decrease in exposure to infection and an improvement in knowledge and skill.

In this chapter, some general strategies for infection prevention, control priorities and methods for risk reduction are discussed, taking into account the patient and service provider's economic, social and home circumstances. In the home environment, it may be necessary to seek cheaper and more innovative methods of infection control to provide the necessary care. Common infection control principles are described, with some examples of their application, though the reader is referred to the previous chapters as well. The goal of this section is to guide home-based caregivers and service providers in developing practical and pioneering infection control programmes, based on the patients' individual needs and available resources. The rewards of a well-designed programme should become measurable in improved care and lowered healthcare costs.

Isolation precautions in home-based care settings mainly consist of:
- washing and disinfecting hands
- using protective clothing and barriers
- maintaining environmental hygiene
- cleaning, disinfecting and sterilising equipment thoroughly
- maintaining a high level of personal hygiene for both the patient and the caregiver.

Infection control measures that can be incorporated into home-based care

Hand hygiene

Skin cannot be sterilised, only disinfected with antiseptic. Micro-organisms on the patients' and caregivers' skin are often associated with infection. Antiseptic hand-washing soap should preferably contain one of the following:

- 2–4% chlorhexidine gluconate (best option)
- 70% ethyl alcohol and/or 70–90% isopropyl alcohol
- 2–3,5% iodophors
- 1,5–3,5% chloroxylenol.

Soap and water are always needed to remove blood or other organic materials from hands and surfaces. Avoid using basins filled with antiseptics or standing water to wash hands in, as they are quickly contaminated and the stagnant water then becomes a source of microbacterial growth. Where no running water is available at all, water can be transported in a container with a screw or tap cap that can be poured by another person or hung up and tipped when necessary. Water in a container should not be kept longer than 24 hours as algae and bacteria will start to grow in it. The patient may need to conserve available water for drinking and cooking, and the caregiver should never use this for washing hands if possible.

Waterless antiseptic hand rubs can be used as a substitute for both patients and staff when soap and running water are not available, and in all cases where caregivers are looking after more than one patient simultaneously, or if hands are not visibly soiled. Waterless hand rubs must contain effective concentrations of antiseptics to check slight contamination. Commercial products usually contain a mixture of antiseptics, alcohol, water and emollients.

Spray bottles containing water and a fresh solution of either vinegar or bleach can be transported relatively easily for hand hygiene, using the following quantities:

- 1 part chlorine (household bleach) in 9 parts boiled, cooled water (to keep it effective change daily to a fresh solution, as much of the free chlorine will evaporate within 24 hours).
- 1 part spirit vinegar in 9 parts boiled, cooled water.

An alternative is wiping hands with a commercial 70% isopropyl alcohol wipe (not commonly recommended as this can severely dry out the hands), or a commercial wipe used for babies' bottoms (this is not as effective and can become very expensive).

Antiseptic hand rubs can be used before and after touching mucous membranes, such as the patient's mouth, non-intact skin or body fluids; or when caring for patients known to be suffering from acute or chronic infections. Always use products with sufficient levels of antiseptic or alcohol-base. Alcohol is less likely to be inactivated in the presence of blood or body fluid than any other antiseptic. 5–10 ml hand disinfectant should be actively rubbed into all the surfaces of the hands and under the fingernails, and left to air-dry. Active friction is necessary to dislodge organisms from the skin during both skin disinfection and hand-washing.

A home-made hand rub can be made with 100 ml 70% alcohol and 2 ml glycerine, propylene glycol or sorbitol and used in small spray/squeeze bottles that are washed, dried and refilled regularly.

Protective clothing

The use of medical supplies can become extremely expensive very quickly in home-based care settings. Often, alternatives must be found in order to maintain a high level of infection control. A few alternatives are shown in the following table:

Table 9.1: Protective clothing alternatives

Item	Replace with
Medical gloves	Reusable kitchen/garden gloves or plastic bags.
Surgical gowns or plastic hospital aprons	A thin plastic raincoat, a plastic refuse bag cut open at the top and sides for the head and arms, or even thin oilskins or rubberised overalls.
Face shields or masks	A scarf or large kerchief tied over the mouth and nose.
Paper or cloth caps	A shower cap, a scarf or large kerchief, or a small plastic bag.
Masks with a splash-guard visor, protective spectacles, goggles or medical face shields	Gardening goggles, welding spectacles or a perspex face shield (e.g. used for home soldering or light welding).
Paper or plastic overshoes	Used, intact plastic shopping bags anchored with sticky tape, elastic bands or string.
Specially bought refuse bags and paper for wrapping discarded items	Recycled plastic shopping bags and recycled newspaper.

Environmental hygiene

All items handled frequently by the patient and caregiver(s), including articles soiled with blood or body fluids, must be washed immediately and kept clean/disinfected regularly enough so that transmission of micro-organisms is unlikely to occur. The environment has the potential of harbouring infectious micro-organisms (e.g. the bacteria that can cause tuberculosis or diarrhoea). Good environmental hygiene includes keeping the patient's surroundings clean and tidy; ensuring that laundry such as bed linen and clothing is washed regularly so that the patient's skin can be kept comfortable, clean and dry; and that meals are prepared, stored and served in an hygienic manner.

Organising patient care and housekeeping responsibilities is important. Careful planning is necessary, especially where there is no one else to help with tasks. Sometimes healthcare staff are required to do some housekeeping tasks for the patient(s) they are looking after. Where possible, the trained caregiver should not do any general housekeeping her/himself, but should keep a discreet eye on what is being done by others in the home. It is part of the home-based caregiver's duties to diplomatically guide and educate household members in correct hygiene and ways to assist. If there is no other choice, compulsory housekeeping tasks should be done after primary patient care has been completed, e.g. making the patient comfortable or feeding him/her is a greater priority than washing the dishes.

Disinfection and sterilisation

NEVER use disinfectants or alcohol-based antiseptics (tinctures) on mucous membranes (the genitalia, mouth, ears or eyes), as they are very irritating. 0,5–4% chlorhexidine gluconate or an idiophor (aqueous iodine mixtures) are better choices, but must only be used under medical supervision.

Instruments and equipment must be disassembled before cleaning and disinfection. Articulated or very intricate instruments that cannot be disassembled must be cleaned well and disinfected in an appropriate manner for the maximum period specified by the instrument manufacturer. The process can usually be accomplished by soaking them in chemical agents or by heat processes (boiling [pasteurisation] or baking/exposure to dry heat in an oven).

The following are prerequisites for disinfection by boiling (pasteurisation):

- Only drinkable or boiled water, or water chlorinated to 0,1%, may be used.
- All items must be clean/washed and rinsed beforehand.
- Items should be completely submerged at all times in the heated water.
- Air must be removed from hollow instruments or tubes during submerging.
- No new item may be added to the load that has already begun to pasteurise/boil.
- Disinfected items must be removed from the container in which the procedure was done with clean washed hands or clean tongs/forceps, without contamination, before the item is allowed to air-dry on a clean surface.
- Only dry items are considered adequately disinfected as the disinfection process continues during the drying stage.
- Clean water must be used for every new cycle of disinfection.

Filtration

This is a low-level method of disinfection. Liquids such as non-municipal water can be filtered through special fluid filters, filter paper or finely woven clean cloth/layers of nylon pantyhose. This is mostly done before disinfecting or boiling water for washing/cooking, to remove visible foreign material. Filters must be changed regularly and kept clean from contagion, e.g. avoid handling with soiled hands.

Boiling

Boiling is done at 100°C for at least 5–20 minutes. Five minutes is usually sufficient time for single items made of metal or hard plastic. Longer times are necessary at high altitudes, for over-crowded containers, and for complex, jointed instruments. Ensure that only items that are completely heat-resistant at a temperature of 100°C are boiled. Always use a clean covered pot on the stove or a hotplate, with items submerged in a container filled with water in a microwave oven, or in a kettle over a fire. Boil gently, as a rolling boil bounces items around, lowers the water level quickly and uses extra fuel. Using a pressure cooker speeds up the process. The disinfection time starts as soon as the coldest part of the load has reached the required temperature and is the actual period during which disinfection takes place (holding /standing time). Air-dry boiled items on a clean surface, or dry items with a dedicated clean towel before storage or use.

The advantages of boiling are that it is a reasonably cheap and reliable disinfection method.

The disadvantages are that it is time consuming and can be expensive. Devices with lumens or channels must be totally submerged and filled with water for the minimum holding time. (Refer to the discussion on heat disinfection and pasteurization on page 160, chapter 5.)

Pasteurisation

This is done with heated water when items are not completely heat-resistant, but will withstand total submersion in heated water, at:

- 65°C for 10 minutes' holding time
- 70°C for 05 minutes' holding time
- 80°C for 01 minute's holding time
- 90°C for 01 second's holding time.

Ensure that only heat-resistant items that can withstand temperatures of 65–90°C are pasteurised. Water is usually boiled and then cooled in the container to the required temperature rather than simply being heated to the required temperature. This ensures that all possible pathogenic micro-organisms in the water are killed. The warmer the water, the quicker the process and the less time needed. Use a clean, covered pot or other heat-resistant container. The water can be heated in a container on the stove, over a fire or in a microwave oven – do this before the cleaned items are added, heated up and the holding time starts, or the hot water is poured over the cleaned items. The temperature must be higher than required, to allow for the cooling effect in both cases. Air-dry on a clean surface, or dry with a dedicated clean towel before storage or use.

The advantages of pasteurisation are that it is a cheap and reliable method.

The disadvantages are that it is time-consuming and can be expensive. Devices with lumens or channels must be totally submerged and filled with water for the minimum holding time.

Baking with dry heat

This is done by exposing a heat-resistant item to direct heat in an oven at 160°C for 60 minutes, or at 180°C for 30 minutes' holding time. Use only for completely heat-resistant items, organic material, powders or material such as cotton or linen, as dry heat may cause discoloration and heat distortion. Dry heat penetrates surfaces less effectively than steam or moist heat, and longer holding times are required. If possible, pre-heat the clean item at the same time as the oven in a washed, closed container and then bake for the required holding time. Cool before use or handling.

The advantages of baking are that it is a cheap and reasonably reliable method.

The disadvantages are that it is time-consuming, can be expensive and dangerous

(containers can explode). This is not a good choice for hollow devices or those with small lumens or channels, as dry heat cannot penetrate the hollows.

Chemical disinfection

(Soaking, mopping or wiping inanimate objects with a chemical agent for between ±10 minutes–10 hours, depending on the manufacturer's guidelines.)

High-level disinfection is achieved when clean items are submerged in a fresh solution of disinfectant such as the aldehydes (e.g. 8% formalin or 2% activated glutaraldehyde, which will sterilise clean surfaces within 6–10 hours of continuous contact) or peracetic acid.

Mid-level disinfection is obtained with chemical agents such as the alcohols (e.g. isopropyl alcohol and methylated spirits), halogens (including 0,5% household chlorine bleach, 1000 ppm free chlorine and povidone iodine), phenols (e.g. carbolic acid), and acetic acid (e.g. spirit vinegar), which can destroy some growing bacteria, most viruses and most fungi, excluding bacterial spores, within 20 minutes.

Low-level disinfection is provided with chemicals that can inhibit or destroy most growing bacteria, and some viruses and fungi after 10 minutes. Some examples include: alcohols, halogens, 0,5% chlorine solution in household bleach, quaternary ammonia compounds, and acetic acid (e.g. spirit vinegar).

The advantages of chemical disinfection are that some chemicals are more readily available and cheaper than others and can be used by most caregivers.

The disadvantages are that not all the chemicals listed are as effective as traditional disinfectants, but will serve the purpose if used as directed in the home. All chemicals are deactivated/neutralised to differing levels by contact with foreign material. Chemicals may leave a residue on the items being disinfected, be corrosive, give off noxious fumes and cause chemical burns if not washed off surfaces that come into contact with skin or mucosa, and can be unreliable if used incorrectly, as contaminated chemicals can become a source of infection themselves. Devices that have lumens or channels must be submerged and filled with disinfectant for the minimum contact time. Micro-organisms can build up a resistance to disinfectants if they are used incorrectly. Chemical disinfection can be very expensive.

Disinfecting drinking water

Add 25 ml clear household bleach to 20 litres of filtered non-municipal water and leave to stand for at least one hour. Water boiled vigorously (a rolling boil) for at least 5 minutes is generally considered safe to drink. In areas where there is no firewood or electricity, filtered water can be poured into a clean, clear plastic bottle and a black plastic bag wrapped around it. The water will be pasteurised to ± 65°C if this container is placed in the direct sun for at least six hours. The water can then be used for drinking and baby feeds. Polluted water or water which contains large amounts of foreign matter must first be filtered through a fine cloth and additional bleach (30 ml for 20 litre water) or chlorine added to reach a 0,1% safety level. Using a container with a narrow neck prevents soiled hands or utensils from contaminating the water, as well as rapid evaporation of the chlorine.

Disinfection by exposure to sunlight

Expose inanimate items as long as possible to sunlight for low-level disinfection. Sunlight as such does not sterilise, but will dry out surfaces. Most pathogenic micro-organisms will not grow on very dry surfaces. Airing bedding and mattresses outside and hanging washing in the sun has long been an accepted home-based disinfection method.

Wounds and broken skin areas can be exposed to sunlight for a short time, either early in the morning or late in the afternoon when the sun is weaker. Skin in wound areas must never be exposed to sunlight for longer than 15 minutes at a time. Avoid sunburn or exposing broken skin areas/rashes that might be aggravated by sunlight or heat. Oncology patients who receive irradiation therapy should never expose their skin to the sun.

Basic nutrition and food management

Flawless kitchen sanitation, careful food handling and a high level of personal hygiene are as necessary when caring for a single patient at home as when catering for a whole hospital filled with patients. Nutrition is extremely important for infection prevention and control. Without good nutrition, the patient is unable to produce antibodies or fight off or cope with infections. Immunosuppressed patients are often prone to diarrhoeal infections, while patients with life-limiting diseases often do not have any appetite, cannot face regular meals or have special dietary requirements, such as low protein or carbohydrate needs.

A terminally ill person may have no appetite, or not need additional nutrition because of a general slowing of all the energy-draining life functions, such as digestion. Available finances may also restrict the availability of food and the choice of meals. Although meals are generally smaller for home-based patients, they may need to be prepared more frequently and stored till needed. Cooking must be done thoroughly – all parts of the food must be heated to the proper temperature, e.g. chicken and pork must be cooked to the bone, without any pink or red meat visible. The holding temperatures of prepared food should be above 60°C or below 8°C, while cooked food that is to be refrigerated must be covered and cooled down as quickly as possible. Warm, perishable food must be cooled before storage, or stored in shallow containers to ensure an internal temperature low enough that bacteria will not thrive or produce toxins. Where no refrigerating facilities are available, food should be prepared as needed or stored in a cooler bag, or in a cool place under a cloth or wire mesh hood.

Ingredients or dishes served raw, such as salad, must be well washed. Raw fruit and vegetables that can be peeled before serving (bananas, oranges, and cabbage) are better than those that are used whole or just washed. In general, the more immunosuppressed the patient is, the fewer raw ingredients should be used in meals, especially if they have been grown in organic soil fertilised with animal manure. In some cases, processed food such as uncooked meat, biltong, cheese or yogurt can cause an infection in a patient with a very low resistance.

Supplemental feeds are generally used for patients who cannot eat, or who do not take in enough nourishment, or may need additional nutrients. These feeds can be commercially prepared or home-made. Home-made feeds often become contaminated with micro-organisms during preparation or use. Even small numbers of micro-organisms can cause severe diarrhoeal infections. Contaminated equipment, faulty preparation or storage processes, poor technique or bad hygiene are often to blame.

Persons who prepare meals or handle food should know :
- The basic principles of personal hygiene and the risk of food-borne disease transmission for each patient they care for.
- The importance of reporting their own diarrhoeal diseases or broken skin areas (especially on hands) to a supervisor, to prevent transmission of the infection to a patient.
- The proper inspection, preparation and storage procedures for all the food they handle.
- The correct operating and cleaning procedures for any equipment used.
- The basic food sanitation and waste management procedures.
- The basic choice of diet for the specific patient they are caring for.

Isolating patients with infections

Physical isolation, in the sense of separating an infectious, dying or very ill patient from his/her supporting family and friends, is a decision that should never be made lightly. Protecting an immunosuppressed patient through strict isolation from all persons who might carry infectious micro-organisms may leave him/her with more **quantity** of life, but without meaningful **quality**. Ideally, the traditional hospice motto is a good one to strive for: 'Putting more life into a patients' days, rather than days into a patient's life'. The balance must be calculated between protection of the exposed and/or susceptible patient as well as the exposed and/or susceptible bystander, and basic infection control. All decisions should be filtered through human concern for the total well-being of the patient, and compassion for the family.

Where patients and family members share beds, the caregiver should evaluate the situation and advise accordingly. Patients with airborne transmissible conditions should not sleep with another person, and should rather use another room. Windows should be kept open for as long as possible and the patient placed so that air flows outwards, away from him or her, and not be trapped in a poorly ventilated area. The environment must be kept as dust-free as possible, as dust traps dried-out mucus and carries infectious particles, such as tuberculosis bacilli nuclei. (Refer also to chapter 4, Housekeeping.)

In cases where isolation may be required, the three pillars of infection control must be taken into account when decisions are made: good patient care practice, occupational health and safety, and environmental hygiene and control. In palliative care practice, when working with patients living with life-limiting diseases, another pillar is added – the wishes and safety of the patient.

Legally notifiable medical conditions contained in Section 45 of the Health Act (Act 63 of 1977)

ICD –10 Class	Code name
A22	Anthrax
A23	Brucellosis
A00	Cholera
A50	Congenital syphilis
A90	Dengue fever
A36	Diphtheria
A98.0	Crimean-Congo haemorrhagic fever
A98.4	Ebola fever
G83	Flaccid paralysis (acute)
A05.0-2	Food poisoning
B96.3	Haemophilus influenzae type B
A96.2	Lassa fever
T56.0	Lead poisoning
A48.1	Legionellosis
A30	Leprosy
B50 – B54	Malaria
A98.3	Marburg fever
B05	Measles
A39.0	Meningococcal infection
O96 – O97	Maternal death
A01.1 – A01.4	Paratyphoid fever
A20	Plague
T60	Poisoning agricultural stock remedies
A80	Poliomyelitis
A82	Rabies
A100 – A102	Rheumatic fever
A92.4	Rift Valley fever
B03	Smallpox
A34 – A35	Tetanus
A33	Tetanus neonatorum
A71	Trachoma
A16.7	Tuberculosis primary
A15	Tuberculosis pulmonary
A15	Tuberculosis of other respiratory organs
A17.0	Tuberculosis of meninges

A18.3	Tuberculosis of intestines, peritoneum
A18.0	Tuberculosis of bones and joints
A18.1	Tuberculosis of genitourinary system
A18.8	Tuberculosis of other organs
A19	Tuberculosis miliary
A15 – A19	Tuberculosis total
A01	Typhoid fever
A75.0	Typhus fever (lice-borne)
A75.2	Typhus fever (flea-borne)
B15	Viral hepatitis fever type A
B16	Viral hepatitis fever type B
B17.8	Viral hepatitis fever non - A non – B
B19	Viral hepatitis unspecified
B15 – B19	Viral hepatitis total
A95	Yellow fever
A37	Whooping cough

Glossary

Aetiology	The causality of disease – how and why a disease occurs.
Agent	A substance, infectious or otherwise, that leads to the production of a specific disease. Is also a synonym for a compound.
Antibiogram	A profile of those antimicrobial agents the cultured micro-organism is sensitive and resistant to.
Antimicrobial agents	Chemical and natural agents that counter the (further) progress of infection in an infected patient in order for the natural resistance mechanisms of the body to recover. The most common antimicrobials are antibiotics (against bacteria), anti-micotics (against fungi) and anti-viral agents.
Antiseptic	A disinfectant which can be applied to living surfaces such as skin, without undue side-effects.
Asepsis	The absence of living pathogenic micro-organisms and/or any infective matter. **Medical asepsis:** The removal or destruction of pathogenic micro-organisms or infected matter through cleaning, pasteurisation, disinfection or sterilisation. **Surgical asepsis:** Protection against infection before, during or after surgery through the use of aseptic or sterile techniques such as surgical hand scrubbing, pre-operative skin disinfection, or sterile theatre procedures.
Aseptic technique	A technique to ensure the absence of infection, both during and after completion of a nursing task or invasive medical intervention, such as the application of sterile or pasteurised devices for wound care, or the obligation to use only clean, freshly mixed disinfectants.
Bactericidal	An agent able to kill bacteria.
Bacteristatic	An agent able to intervene with or inhibit bacterial growth.
Barrier nursing	The use of measures including protective clothing, patient isolation, cleaning, disinfecting and sterilisation to prevent the transmission of infectious agents from an infected patient to the staff/patients/ environment.
Biohazard	Matter or items that contain living micro-organisms that might be/are hazardous to a handler's health.
Bioload/bioburden	The load of living micro-organisms on a surface, such as clothing or bed linen.
Carrier	A person or animal harbouring a specific infectious agent that serves as a source of infection without having the discernable clinical disease. Carriers may act as asymptomatic, transient or chronic carriers.
Chain of infection	The process of infection, requiring a source, a route of transmission, and a new susceptible host.
Chemotherapy	Treatment of a condition with chemical agents.
Cleaning	The physical removal of soiling/contamination such as organic matter from surfaces, rendering them safe for use.

Colonisation	The presence, without entry or multiplication, of micro-organisms on a susceptible surface.
Commensal	Micro-organism(s) normally found on a healthy person.
Communicable disease	An illness arising from transmission of a specific infective agent, or its products, from person-to-person, person-to-animal-to-person, or person-to-environment-to-person.
Community-acquired infection	Signs and symptoms of infection that were present when the patient was admitted to the hospital/healthcare facility.
Contact	A person or animal associated with an infected person, animal or environment in such a manner that infection may have been transmitted.
Contamination	The presence of an infectious agent on a living or non-living surface, often invisible to the naked eye.
Disinfectant	An agent that destroys or inhibits disease-causing micro-organisms.
Disinfection	The removal or inactivation of vegetative micro-organisms from surfaces, but not necessarily the removal of bacterial spores.
Endogenous infection	An infection arising due to contamination from the patient's own body.
Exogenous infection	An infection arising due to contamination from a source outside the patient's body.
Exposure	Circumstances potentially leading to infection.
Fomites	Any articles or substances other than food that may transmit infectious micro-organisms.
Fumigation	A process by which insects and micro-organisms are destroyed with gaseous agents.
Hand hygiene	Consists of hand-washing (with soap and running water) and hand disinfection (the application of an appropriate antiseptic to the skin).
Healthcare institutions Health institutions Healthcare facilities Patient-care facilities/institutions	Permanent or transitory places where primary, secondary and tertiary patient care is given.
Healthcare practitioners Healthcare worker Healthcare personnel	Persons responsible for patient care.
Hospital-acquired infection (HAI)	Infection that presents within 48 hours of hospitalisation, of which there were no signs and symptoms before admittance.
Hydrophilic	Used for wound dressings that contain or encourage a moist wound-healing atmosphere.
Hydrophobic	Wound dressings that repel moistness.
Host	A person or animal that permanently or transiently harbours an infectious agent.
Immunity	Possessing specific protective antibodies or cellular immunity due to a previous infection or immunisation. Immunity is relative; an ordinarily effective resistance may be overwhelmed by an excessive dose of the infectious agent or via an unusual portal of entry as well as by immunosuppressive chemo-therapy or concurrent disease.
Incubation period	The time interval between exposure to an infectious agent and appearance of the first sign or symptom of the disease in question.

Infected person	A person who harbours an infectious agent and manifests the disease, or has inapparent infection.
Infection control	The establishment and maintenance of a safe environment for patients and staff members, providing the highest level of protection with the available resources, based on scientific principles.
Infection	The entry and development or multiplication of an infectious agent in the body of the host, leading to a clinical host reaction.
Infectious person	A person from whom the infectious agent can be naturally acquired.
Infestation	The presence, entry, development and reproduction of arthropods in the environment, in animals, on the body or in the clothes of a person.
Isolation	Separation, for the period of communicability, of infected persons from other persons to prevent the direct or indirect transfer of infection.
MRSA	Multi drug resistant *Staphylococcus aureus*.
MRSE	Multi drug resistant *Staphylococcus epidermidis*.
Nosocomial infection	An infection originating in a medical facility (hospital acquired infection), without any sign and symptom of it being present on admittance.
Opportunistic pathogen	A micro-organism that normally exists in symbiosis with its environment, that may cause infection when moved to another, more susceptible environment.
Occupationally acquired infection	An infection that is acquired while at work during normal or routine patient care tasks, without any sign or symptom of it being present during the period before the work is done/contact is made with a patient.
Pasteurisation	The use of moist heat at 65–90 ºC to destroy vegetative micro-organisms.
Pathogen	A micro-organism with the ability to cause illness in a susceptible host.
Personal hygiene	Individual protective measures that promote health and combat the spread of infection.
Resistance	The sum total of body mechanisms that interpose barriers to the invasion or multiplication of infectious agents or damage by their toxic products.
Service provider	A private, parastatal, welfare or non-governmental organisation rendering a service to patients in their own homes or in an in-patient unit, by way of lay or trained healthcare staff.
Soiling (pollution)	The visible presence of dirt or offensive matter on a living or non-living surface that should be clean.
Source of infection	The person, object, animal or substance from which an infectious agent passes directly to a host. The source may be living or non-living.
Spores	A method of ensuring the micro-organism's continued existence when living conditions become hostile, e.g. drying or starvation. Example: a bacteria's genetic material is encased in a capsule, with loss of any non-essential protein and structures. In this format, the genetic material can survive for long periods until conditions become more conducive to proliferation and germination takes place again.
Sterilisation	The total eradication of all living micro-organisms and spores.
Strategy	A process used to prevent or manage problems.
Susceptibility	A person or animal without sufficient resistance to a specific pathogen to counter the transmission and establishment of infection.

Surgically clean	Washed clean with soap and water, and safe to use. Also used to refer to aseptically scrubbed hands.
Terminal disinfection	The process of rendering the personal possessions and immediate physical environment of a patient free from the possibility of transmitting infection after the patient has been removed or has ceased to be a source of infection or after isolation practises have been discontinued.
Tincture	An antiseptic or disinfectant solution with alcohol as base, e.g. tincture of iodine.
Topical antiseptic agent	Antiseptics (disinfectants compatible with living tissue) that are applied to the skin's surface, e.g. disinfectant hand rubs that usually contain a minimum of emollient and alcohol (plus another disinfectant ingredient at times).
Transmission of infection	The mechanism by which a susceptible host is exposed to an infectious agent, including direct and indirect contact (air, vector and droplet transmission).
VRE	Vancomycin resistant *Enterococcus*.
Virulence	The degree to which micro-organisms are able to cause disease.
Waste	**Household:** Waste that contains no potential or definite infectious ingredients, e.g. disposable paper, plastic, metal bottle caps, or kitchen refuse. Can be disposed of in a municipal landfill.
	Medical: Waste that contains disposable items that have been in contact with a patient's blood or body fluids, e.g. wound dressings, paper tissues, incontinence nappies. Should be incinerated, decontaminated, sterilised or buried.
	Sharps: Disposable glass ampoules, vials or bottles; lancets; blood glucose pricks; scalpel blades that have been in contact with blood or body fluids as well as any other items that can potentially break, abrade, cut or damage a waste handler's skin or tissues. Should be incinerated, decontaminated, sterilised or buried deeply.

Index of sources

Anderson, K.N., Anderson, L.E. and Glanze, W.D. 1998. *Mosby's Medical, Nursing, and Allied Health Dictionary.* Fourth edition. St. Louis: Mosby Company.

Anderson, K.N. and Anderson, L.E. 1990. *Mosby's Pocket Dictionary of Medicine, Nursing, and Allied Health.* St. Louis: D.V. Mosby Company.

APIC *Text of Infection Control and Epidemiology*, Volume 1 and 2. 2000. APIC Inc.: Washington.

Ayliffe, G.A.J., Collins, B.J. and Taylor, L.J. 1991. *Hospital-acquired infection: Principles and Prevention:* Second edition. Surrey: Butterworth-Heinemann.

Bedryfsgesondheid [s.a.]. *Bedryfsgesondheidsgevare: Aansteeklike siektes.* Aanhangsel IV. Bloemfontein: Universitas/Nasionale Hospitale 1996, pp. 1–5.

Benenson, A.S. (ed.). 1995. *Control of communicable diseases in man.* Sixteenth edition. Washington: American Public Health Association.

Bennett, J V and Brachman, P S, (eds.). 1998. *Hospital Infections.* Fourth edition, Lippincott-Raven Publishers: Philadelphia.

Berkow, R. (ed.). 1982. *The MERCK Manual of Diagnosis and Therapy.* Rahway: MERCK and Co., Inc.

Brink, A.J. et al. 2004. *Woordeboek van Afrikaanse Geneeskundeterme.* Sewende druk. Kaapstad: Pharos Bpk.

Coates, D. 1992. A comparison of the methods used in a UK hospital to decontaminate spills of body fluids. Nursing RSA Verpleging, Vol. 7, No. 5, pp. 45–46.

Coates, D. 1992. Disinfectants and spills of body fluid. *Nursing RSA Verpleging*, Vol. 7, No. 6, pp. 25–27.

Collins, T.F.B. 1992. AIDS and TB: Overlooked dimension. *Nursing RSA Verpleging*, Vol. 7, No. 6, pp. 25–27.

Church, D. February 2000. Changes in Procedure for Culture of Vascular Catheter Tips and Implanted Devices. http://www.crha-health.ab.ca/clin/cme/microbio.htm Calgary Laboratory Services Microbiology Newsletter, February 2000, pp. 1–2. [Retrieval date 27 09 2004]

Dalgety, Y. 1992. Infection control in a trauma unit. *Nursing RSA Verpleging*, Vol. 7, No. 5, pp. 37–38.

Davis, J. 1992. Blood-borne pathogens: Safety for the healthcare worker. *Nursing RSA Verpleging*, vol. 7, No. 9, No. 9, pp. 23–26.

Departement van Nasionale Gesondheid en Bevolkingsontwikkeling. 1992. *Annexure to the proposed regulations of communicable diseases – to replace Regulation R2438 of 30.10.87*, pp. 51–54.

Dictionary Unit for South African English. 2002. *South African Concise Oxford Dictionary.*

Die Stad Bloemfontein [s.a.]. *Lekehandleiding: Aansteeklike siektes; aanmeldbare siektes; skooluitsluiting*, pp. 1–14.

Evian, C. 2001. *Primary AIDS care.* Third edition. Houghton: JACANA Publishers.

Forder, A.A. 1992. The costs of hospital-associated infection in South Africa. *Nursing RSA Verpleging*, Vol. 7, No. 10, 20–22.

Forder, A.A. 1992. The re-use of single-use medical devices. *Nursing RSA Verpleging*, Vol. 7, No. 5, pp. 33–36.

Garner, J.S. and Simmons, B.P. [s.a.]. *CDC guideline for isolation precautions in hospitals.* Atlanta, Georgia: U.S. Department of Health and Human Services.

Glass, C.A. and Grap, M.J. 1995. Ten tips for safer suctioning. *American Journal of*

Nursing, May 1995, pp. 51–53.

Gould, D. 1987. *Infection and patient care: a guide for nurses.* London: Heinemann Nursing.

Gould, D. 1995. Hand decontamination: Nurses' opinions and practices. *Nursing Times*, Vol. 91, no. 17, pp. 42–45.

Greenwood, D; Slack, R. and Peutherer, J. (eds.). 1998. *Medical Microbiology – A guide to microbial infections: Pathogenesis, Immunity, Laboratory Diagnosis and Control.* Fifteenth edition. London: ELST with Churchill Livingstone.

Gruendermann, B.J. 1992. Handwashing and gloves. *Nursing RSA Verpleging*, vol. 7, no. 5, p. 46.

Gruendermann, B.J. 1992. Universal precautions in the operating room. *Nursing RSA Verpleging*, vol. 7, No. 5, pp. 41.

Gustaffson, G. and Moodley, M. 1992. Infection control in a hospital creche. *Nursing RSA Verpleging*, Vol. 7, No. 8, pp. 18-20.

Heaton, W.H. and Thayer, N.L. 1991. *Infection control program: Policy and procedure manual.* Baltimore: National Health Publishing.

Heenan, A. 1990. Indications for long-term catheterisation. *Nursing Times*, Vol. 86, No. 14, pp. 7071.

Heenan, A. 1992. Handwashing practices. *Nursing Times*, Vol, 88, No. 34, p. 70.

Kennedy, J., et.al.; Selection and use of disinfectants. http:// ianrpubs.unl.edu/animal disease/g1410.htm retrieval date 03.03.2004

Kolff, C.A. and Sánchez, R. 1979. *Handbook for infectious disease management.* Menlo Park, California: Addison-Wesley Publishing Company.

Lawrence, C. 1992. Testing alcohol wipes. *Nursing Times*, Vol. 88, No. 34, pp. 63–66.

Maartens, G. 1994. The early stages of HIV infection: Clinical features and management. *Modern medicine of South Africa*, Vol. 19, No. 7, pp. 39–44.

Marais, H. 1992. Malaria: Nursing management. *Nursing RSA Verpleging*, Vol. 7, No. 5, p. 44.

Mayet, F.M. 1992. Management of sharps injuries. *Nursing RSA Verpleging*, Vol. 7, No. 5, pp. 30–32.

McCarthy, T.M. 1992. Antiseptics and disinfectants – what are they? *Nursing RSA Verpleging*, Vol. 7, No. 5, p. 46.

Monteagudo, F.S.E., Havlik, I. and Hempelman, E. 1992. Malaria: Symptoms, signs and treatment. *Nursing RSA Verpleging*, Vol. 7, No. 5, p.44.

Morgan, D. (ed.). 1989. *Infection control: The British Medical Association Guide.* London: Edward Arnold.

Morgan, D.A. 1992. Wound management. *Nursing RSA Verpleging*, Vol. 7, No. 9, pp. 17–19.

Mulder, M. (ed.). 1999. *Practical guide for general nursing science, part 2.* Cape Town: Maskew Miller Longman.

Mulder, M, N Small, Y Botma, L Ziady, J MacKenzie. 2002. *Basic principles of wound care.* Cape Town: Pearson Education South Africa

Muller, M. 1992. Legal aspects in the nursing of patients with infectious diseases. *Nursing RSA Verpleging*, Vol. 7, No. 5, p. 47.

Odendaal, F.F. (hoofred.). (et al.) 1984. *Verklarende handwoordeboek van die Afrikaanse taal.* Tweede uitgawe. Johannesburg: PERSKOR Uitgewery.

OEHS WEB. Biosafety Program Home Page. *Summary and comparison of liquid disinfectants.* http://keats.admin.virginia.edu/bio/disinfectant-summary.html retrieval date 03. 03. 2004

Palmer, M.B. 1984. *Infection control: a policy and procedure manual.* Philadelphia: W.B. Saunders Company.

Park, C. 1992. Meningococcal meningitis nursing management. *Nursing RSA Verpleging*, Vol. 7, No. 5, pp. 42.

Parkin, J.M. and Peters, B.S. 1991. *Differential diagnosis in AIDS – a colour guide.* Switzerland: Wolfe Publishing Ltd.

Pearse, J. 1992. Infection control of enteral feeds. *Nursing RSA Verpleging*, Vol. 7, No. 7, pp 28–31.

Pearse, J. 1992. Nursing management of patient with hepatitis A and B. *Nursing RSA Verpleging*, Vol. 7, No. 5, pp. 28-29.

Pearse, J. 1997. *Infection Control Manual.* Jacana Publishers : Johannesburg.

Pearse, J. and Mabuse, D. 1992. The infection control nursing management of a patient with acute tuberculosis. *Nursing RSA Verpleging*, Vol. 7, No. 5, p. 42.

Pheipher, J A, ed. (et.al.). 1998. *APIC Text of Infection Control and Epidemiology*, Volume 1 (1998) APIC Inc.: Washington.

Rawson, D. 2004. *The Basics of Surgical Mask Selection.* www.infectioncontroltoday.com/articles/331feat2.html. Retrieval date 25.10.2004

Reese, R E and Betts, R F. 1996. *A Practical Approach to Infectious Diseases.* Fourth edition. Little, Brown and Company: Boston.

Roberts, M.T.M. Common Viral Infections. *Curriculum II.* September 2004/Update. pp.12–17.

Ryan, K J. (ed.). 1990. *Sherris Medical Microbiology.* 3rd edition. Appleton-Lange: Connecticut.

Seymour, J. 1995. Uniforms: Making them work for you. *Nursing Times*, Vol. 91, No. 19, pp. 47–48.

Simms, R. and Moss, V. 1991. *Terminal care for people with AIDS.* MIDMAY Mission Hospital. London: Edward Arnold.

Strauss, S.A. 1984. *Legal handbook for nurses and health personnel.* Fifth edition. Cape Town: King Edward VII Trust.

Suid-Afrika (Republiek). Departement van Statistiek [s.a.]. *Handleiding: Statistiese indeling van siektes, beserings en die dood.* Pretoria: Staatsdrukker.

Teuwen, D. 1992. Viral hepatitis: The whole spectrum. *Nursing RSA Verpleging*, Vol. 7, No. 5, p. 45.

Teuwen, D.J. and Cattell, S.F. 1992. Infection control and sexually transmitted diseases. *Nursing RSA Verpleging*, Vol. 7, No. 5, p. 44.

Tulloch, S. (ed.). 1993. *Reader's Digest Oxford Complete Wordfinder.* London: Reader's Digest Association Limited.

Turner, T. 1995. Life-saving chore. *Nursing Times*, Vol. 91, No. 07, p. 20.

Uys, L. and Cameron, S. 2003. *Home-Based HIV/AIDS Care.* Cape Town: Oxford University Press.

Van den Berg, R.H. en Viljoen, M.J. (red.). 1989. *Oordraagbare siektes: 'n Verpleegkundige perspektief.* Pretoria: De Jager-HAUM Uitgewers.

Verschoor, T; Fick, G H; Jansen, R-M; Viljoen, DJ. 1996. *Verpleegkunde en die Reg.* Kenwyn: Juta en Kie.

Voss, A. and Wallrauch, M.D. 1995. Scabies outbreak among hospital health workers. *Nursing Times*, Vol. 91, No. 17.

Weinstein, S. 1992. Urinary tract infections. *Nursing RSA Verpleging*, Vol. 7, No. 5, p. 44.

Wentzel, R.P. (ed.). 1987. *Prevention and control of nosocomial infections.* Baltimore: Williams and Wilkins.

West, K. 1992. Assesing the risks. *Emergency*, Vol. 24, No. 3, pp. 30–33.

Williams, W.W. *CDC guideline for infection control in hospital personnel.* Atlanta, Georgia: U.S. Department of Health and Human Services.

Wilson, J. 2000. *Clinical Microbiology – An introduction for Healthcare professionals.* Eighth edition. Edinburgh: Baillière Tindall.

Worsley, M. 1992. Handwashing – why is it important? *Nursing RSA Verpleging*, Vol. 7, No. 5, p. 46.

Worsley, M. 1992. Urinary tract infection. *Nursing RSA Verpleging*, Vol. 7, No. 5, p. 45.

Ziady, L.E. 1994. Praktiese Handleiding Deel II: Infeksiebeheer manuskrip, Infeksiebeheer Afdeling Universitas/Nasionale Hospitale, Bloemfontein.

Ziady, L.E.; N. Small, and A.M.J. Louis. 1997. *Infection Control Rapid Reference.* Pretoria: Kagiso Tertiary Publishers.

Ziady, L.E., Editorial: Let's talk rubbish – the management of hospital waste. *Infection Control Journal of Southern Africa.* September 1997, 2(2): 3–7.

Index

100669

785
DH 9.10

Marian Cox

COLEG CYMUNEDOL ABERGELE
ABERGELE COMMUNITY COLLEGE
CANOLFAN ADNODDAU DYSGU
LEARNING RESOURCE CENTRE
FFON/TEL 01745 828 100
Return on or before the last date stamped below.

Staff loan only

Pride and Prejudice

Jane Austen

LITERATURE

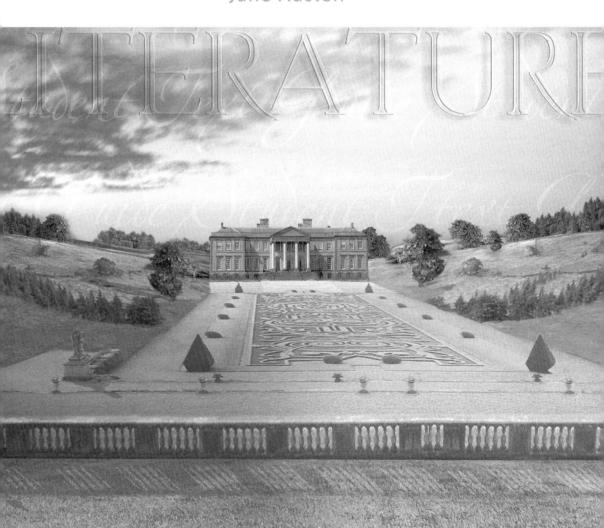

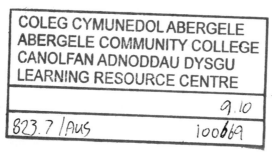

COLEG CYMUNEDOL ABERGELE
ABERGELE COMMUNITY COLLEGE
CANOLFAN ADNODDAU DYSGU
LEARNING RESOURCE CENTRE

9.10

823.7 / Aus   100669

Philip Allan Updates, an imprint of Hodder Education, an Hachette UK Company, Market Place, Deddington, Oxfordshire OX15 0SE

Orders
Bookpoint Ltd, 130 Milton Park, Abingdon, Oxfordshire, OX14 4SB
tel: 01235 827720
fax: 01235 400454
e-mail: uk.orders@bookpoint.co.uk
Lines are open 9.00 a.m.–5.00 p.m., Monday to Saturday, with a 24-hour message answering service. You can also order through the Philip Allan Updates website: www.philipallan.co.uk

© Philip Allan Updates 2009

ISBN 978-0-340-96577-1

First printed 2009

Impression number   5   4   3   2

Year   2014   2013   2012   2011   2010   2009

All rights reserved; no part of this publication may be reproduced, stored in a retrieval system, or transmitted, in any form or by any means, electronic, mechanical, photocopying, recording or otherwise without either the prior written permission of Philip Allan Updates or a licence permitting restricted copying in the United Kingdom issued by the Copyright Licensing Agency Ltd, Saffron House, 6–10 Kirby Street, London EC1N 8TS.

In all cases we have attempted to trace and credit copyright owners of material used.

Printed in Malta

Environmental information
Hachette UK's policy is to use papers that are natural, renewable and recyclable products and made from wood grown in sustainable forests. The logging and manufacturing processes are expected to conform to the environmental regulations of the country of origin.